Urgent Care Guide in Otolaryngology
A 5-step approach

Ricardo Persaud | Sean Fang | Maha Khan |
Eugene Wong | Yogesh Bhatt

Foreword by **Professor Ram Dhillon** *FRCS,*
Consultant ENT Surgeon

1st Edition 2014

Ricardo A P Persaud

MBBS MPhil FRCS ORL HNS (Eng) CCT Otol. (UK)
Consultant ENT Surgeon (Locum)
University Hospitals of Leicester
Leicester Royal Infirmary
United Kingdom

Sean Fang

MB ChB MRCS (ENT)
Core Surgical Trainee
Leeds Teaching Hospitals
Yorkshire and Humber Deanery

Maha Khan

MBChB MRCS (ENT)
Core Surgical Trainee
Manchester
North West Rotation
United Kingdom

Eugene Wong

MBChB MRCS (Gen) MRCS (ENT)
Research Fellow in Otolaryngology
Common Cold Centre and Healthcare Clinical Trials
Cardiff School of Biosciences
Cardiff University
United Kingdom

Yogesh M Bhatt

MBChB (Hons), BSc (Hons), FRCS ORL-HNS (Ed)
ST8 Higher Surgical Trainee
Salford Royal Hospital NHS Foundation Trust
North West Deanery
United Kingdom

First published 2014 by FASTPRINT PUBLISHING
Peterborough, England.

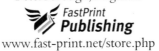

www.fast-print.net/store.php

URGENT CARE GUIDE IN OTOLARYNGOLOGY
A 5-STEP APPROACH
Copyright © Ricardo Persaud, Sean Fang, Maha Khan,
Eugene Wong & Yogesh Bhatt 2014

The right of Ricardo Persaud, Sean Fang, Maha Khan, Eugene Wong &
Yogesh Bhatt to be identified as the authors of this work has
been asserted by them in accordance with the Copyright, Designs and
Patents Act 1988 and any subsequent amendments thereto.

A catalogue record for this book is available from the British Library

ISBN 978-178035-759-1

An environmentally friendly book printed and bound in England by
www.printondemand-worldwide.com

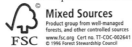

Mixed Sources
Product group from well-managed
forests, and other controlled sources
www.fsc.org Cert no. TT-COC-002641
© 1996 Forest Stewardship Council
FSC

PEFC Certified
This product is
from sustainably
managed forests
and controlled
sources
www.pefc.org
PEFC
PEFC/16-33-415

This book is made entirely of chain-of-custody materials

Urgent Care Guide in Otolaryngology
A 5-step Approach

CONTENTS

- Preface   9
- Foreword   11
- Acknowledgements   15
- Dedications   17

CHAPTER 1: Ear   **19**

1.1   Foreign body in the ear   19
1.2   Otitis externa   23
1.3   Acute otitis media (AOM)   27
1.4   Acute mastoiditis   32
1.5   Facial nerve palsy (lower motor neurone)   35
1.6   Sudden sensori-neural hearing loss (SSNHL) 41
1.7   Acute vertigo   45
1.8   Pinna laceration and haematoma auris   50
1.9   Temporal bone fracture (inc CSF leak)   54
1.10 Infected pre-auricular sinus   58
1.11 Perichondritis of the external ear   61
1.12 Relapsing polychondritis   63
1.13 Furunculosis   65
1.14 Traumatic perforation of tympanic membrane
      (inc NAI)   67
1.15 Necrotising otitis externa (NOE)   70

CHAPTER 2: Nose and Bronchus   **72**

2.1   Foreign body in nose (inc rhinolith)   72
2.2   Foreign body in bronchus (inc speaking valve) 76
2.3   Epistaxis anterior   82

2.4   Epistaxis posterior   88
2.5   Epistaxis in special conditions   92
2.6   Fractured nose   98
2.7   Septal haematoma   102
2.8   Acute rhinosinusitis (ARS)   105
2.9   Peri-orbital cellulitis   108
2.10 Pott's puffy tumour   112
2.11 CSF rhinorhoea   115
2.12 Mucormycosis   118
2.13 Bilateral choanal atresia   121
2.14 Neonatal rhinitis   126

CHAPTER 3: Throat and Oesophagus   128

3.1   Food bolus in oesophagus   128
3.2   Foreign body in the pharynx or oesophagus   131
3.3   Tonsillitis   134
3.4   Quinsy (peritonsillar abscess) and peritonsillar
      cellulitis   138
3.5   Acute epiglottis   142
3.6   Croup (laryngotracheobronchitis)   145
3.7   Stridor in adults   147
3.8   Vincent's angina   150
3.9   Angio-oedema   152
3.10 Caustic ingestion   154

CHAPTER 4: Neck and Head   156

4.1   Neck trauma   156
4.2   Superficial neck abscess   162
4.3   Deep neck space infection   165
4.4   Ludwig's angina   171
4.5   Lemierre's disease (human necrobacillosis)   174
4.6   Cavernous sinus thrombosis (CST)   176
4.7   Sigmoid sinus thrombosis   178
4.8   Erysipelas   182

4.9   Cervical necrotizing fasciitis   184

CHAPTER 5: Complications of treatment   187

5.1   Adenotonsillectomy haemorrhage (shock)   187
5.2   Oesophageal perforation   190
5.3   Post thyroidectomy haematoma   193
5.4   Hypocalcaemia following total thyroidectomy   195
5.5   Facial nerve palsy after tympanomastoid surgery   197
5.6   Tracheoinnominate fistula   199
5.7   Chyle leak   203
5.8   Laryngectomy speech valve leak   206
5.9   Radiation mucocitis   209
5.10   Bismuth Iodoform Paraffin Paste (BIPP) reaction   211
5.11   Drug induced hearing loss   214
5.12   BAHA infection   217
5.13   Cochlear implant infection   222
5.14   Carotid blowout   225

Glossary   228

Preface

The specialty of Otolaryngology is often inadequately covered at medical schools and as a result many new doctors find it an intimidating field at the start of their initial ENT placement. We have all been through the daunting experiences of our first ENT on-call shift, dealing with an ENT emergency on the ward or in the Emergency Department. With these shortcomings in mind, we decided to put together this book, which provides a structured framework to deal with any clinical case.

Whilst acknowledging the myriad of textbooks available for ENT, we are unaware of any guide that provides clear succinct information for the new junior doctor on how to deal with conditions requiring urgent care. This book provides a simple logical 5-step approach to the management of ENT emergency and semi-emergency disorders, including acute complications of treatment. The 5 steps of management are history, examination, investigation, treatment and follow-up. We have presented only the important information required to understand and deal with the problem; the most important 'treatment' section is highlighted in the urgent care colour Orange. Therefore, armed with this latest ENT TZAR guidebook, those new to ENT can be confident that they can deal with most, if not all, urgent care challenges in Otolaryngology practice.

It may be worth noting that all the advice given here represents schema to allow you to familiarise yourself with assessing and treating urgent ENT cases only. It is not intended to be a didactic instructive guide or textbook. Furthermore local hospital protocols should be followed wherever appropriate. We hope that you enjoy this book as much as we enjoyed putting it together.

Ricardo Persaud
Sean Fang
Maha Khan
Eugene Wong
Yogesh Bhatt

January 2014

Foreword

It gives me great pleasure to write the foreword for this new urgent care book aimed at all who deal with ENT patients. With every change over of junior doctors there is always the palpable sense of anxiety in those who are new to this field. I can only sympathise with their apprehension as it is a very steep learning curve, with juniors required to learn new clinical knowledge and practical skills on a system of the body that is infrequently dealt with during medical school and foundation training.

The unique 5 step approach the authors have used is a fantastic way of cutting out the chaff and getting straight to the point. There is no long-winded woolly text, only the salient points pertaining to management of each acute condition are presented. Whether you are a new surgical trainee facing your first on-call or an emergency doctor seeing your first ENT patient, this guidebook gives you the tools to manage urgent ENT problems with confidence. I am sure that this book will raise the standard of acute ENT care because of its no nonsense format.

Professor Ram Dhillon FRCS
Consultant ENT Surgeon, Northwick Park Hospital,
London, UK.
Visiting Professor, Middlesex University
Clinical Director, Rila Institute of Health Sciences,
London.

January 2014

"A stitch in time saves nine"

Acknowledgements

We would like to acknowledge the excellent contributions of Gada Yasin and Zei-Wei Li. Many thanks to Anusha Bala for her comments on the manuscript and for some of the clinical photographs. We are also grateful to Alexander Yao for his advice on the organisation of the information and to Sharon Sankey for the hours spent reformatting the manuscript. Special thanks to Ffion Davies, Shradha Gupta, Shalini Patiar and Bindy Sahota for their generous editorial help.

To all the ambassadors of ENT TZAR
Past, Present and Future

Chapter 1

Ear

1.1 FOREIGN BODY IN THE EAR

1 History

- Nature of the foreign body (FB) i.e. organic, non-organic, caustic
- Duration of insertion
- Associated bleeding, pain, hearing loss

2 Examination

- Otoscopy to confirm FB and any associated trauma
- Check opposite ear

3 Investigation(s)

- Not required

4 Treatment

- Foreign body should only be removed with the trust of the patient and by a trained individual ideally under oto-microscopic guidance.
- Children will not allow multiple attempts and poor technique may lead to an unnecessary general anaesthetic (GA).
- Foreign body may be suctioned out (esp. spherical objects) or pulled out using a wax hook or crocodile forceps.
- Button batteries require **urgent** removal.
- Insects can be drowned with olive oil before removal
- Avoid irrigating organic FB – they may swell due to hydrophilic nature.

5 Follow-up and additional information

- If FB is non-caustic it may be removed by an experienced colleague in the outpatient department (OPD) ideally <2/52
- No follow up is required if no trauma to external auditory canal (EAC) or tympanic membrane (TM).
- Advise water precautions and review in clinic in <3/52 if evidence of canal or drum trauma.

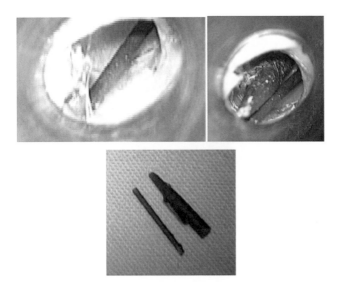

Figures 1.1a Foreign bodies (pencil lead) in the left and right ear canals of a child.

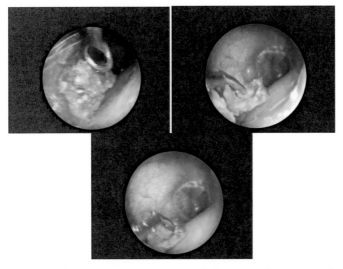

Figure 1.1b Endoscopic removal of FB from the ear canal with a Jobson Horne probe used as a rake.

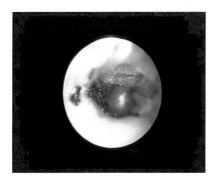

Figure 1.1c Tick in the ear canal.

1.2 OTITIS EXTERNA

1 History

- Discharge
- Otalgia
- Pruritis
- +/- Hearing loss
- Risk factors include cotton-tip user, hearing aid, swimmer, diabetic, immunosuppressed, skin condition eg eczema, psoriasis.

2 Examination

- Inspect for pinna or facial involvement – may require admission for intravenous (IV) antibiotic therapy.
- Assess facial nerve function – is a manifestation of skull-base osteomyelitis (rare).
- Otoscopy to confirm diagnosis, assess canal patency and presence of drum perforation.
- Infection localised to the outer hair bearing part of the canal may represent furunculosis.

3 Investigation(s)

- Microbiological swab for culture and sensitivity of bacteria +/- fungi

- Discuss with senior if facial palsy – requires inpatient investigation and treatment.

4 Treatment

- Microbiological swab for culture and sensitivity of bacteria +/- fungi.
- Strict water precautions and topical therapy (eg sofradex 3drops tds 10/7) are the cornerstones of treatment.
- Micro-otoscopy with suction of canal debris may also be essential, especially for refractory cases.
- If canal is narrowed, use a Pope wick to aid drop delivery into the deep canal (must be removed in 72hrs).
- Consider systemic antibiotics if pinna or facial cellulitis is present.
- Consider admission for analgesia if necessary or if spreading infection or suspicion of necrotising otitis externa eg facial nerve palsy or canal granulations with disproportionate pain.
- Otomycosis requires topical antifungal medication for at least 2 weeks beyond the resolution of clinical signs to eradicate spores.
- Steroid ointments with antibiotic (eg Betnovate-C) are also available for insertion into the ear canal.

5 Follow-up and additional information

- Water precautions can be achieved by using cotton

wool and Vaseline to the conchal bowl in shower etc. Avoid hearing aids, cotton-tips.

- Review refractory cases in one week to monitor effectiveness of treatment
- If a Pope wick has been inserted review in 2-3 days to remove wick and replace if gross canal oedema persists
- Self removal of pope wick can be facilitated by adding a silk suture to the end and taping the thread to the face until time for removal
- Persistent foul smelling otorrhoea >6/52 suggests cholesteatoma until proven otherwise.

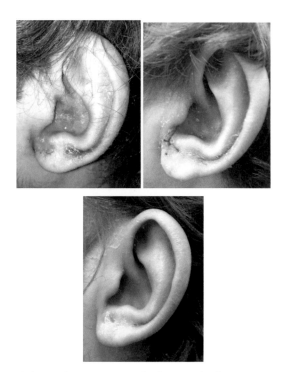

Figures 1.2a-c Otitis externa before and after treatment with antibiotic ear drops (locorten vioform) and topical steroid (Synalar) ointment.

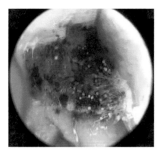

Figure 1.2d Otomycosis of the external ear canal.

1.3 ACUTE OTITIS MEDIA (AOM)

1 History

- Often preceded by upper respiratory tract infection (URTI).
- Progressive otalgia often followed by large volume thin ear discharge with the resolution of otalgia following drum perforation
- Hearing loss
- Systemic symptoms including meningism
- Immunosuppression or h/o previous complications of AOM
- Cochlear implant – these cases must be discussed with senior ENT trainee.

2 Examination

- Otoscopy shows a inflamed, bulging red tympanic membrane
- Mucopurulent discharge may be present if there is a perforation of the TM
- Secondary otitis externa may also be present
- Exclude signs of complications including post-auricular fluctuance, meningism, facial palsy.

3 Investigation(s)

- Swab for MC+S if refractory to initial therapy or systemic signs.

4 Treatment

- Analgesia and antipyretics for first 72 hours (may be viral aetiology) unless systemically unwell, active/prior complications, immunosuppression or bilateral otorrhoea in the under 2yrs-old
- Antibiotics after 72 hours if no improvement – e.g. co-amoxiclav 25mg/kg/day for one week (to cover *haemophilus influenza*, *streptococcus sp.* and *moraxella catarrhalis)*
- Topical therapy may treat secondary otitis externa but should be limited to 10/7 if drum perforation possible
- Admit if signs of severe illness or complications including mastoid collection, meningism or gross malaise.
- Myringotomy is reserved for AOM with complications or to relieve drug refractory pain.
- Any patient with AOM and cochlear implant must be discussed with a senior ENT colleague.

5 Follow-up and additional information

- Simple AOM does not require follow-up.

- Acute otitis media (AOM) should be distinguished from otitis media with effusion (OME or glue ear) which describes non-purulent fluid behind an intact tympanic membrane and is often asymptomatic.

- Complications of AOM may be classified as those that involve the temporal bone, intracranial and extracranial regions.

- Long-term sequelae of AOM include non-suppurative middle ear effusion, high frequency sensorneural hearing loss, tympanic membrane perforation, adhesions, tympanosclerosis and erosion of the ossicular chain.

- Recurrent otorrhoea for >6/52 without resolution raises the suspicion of established drum perforation by cholesteatoma and therefore requires ENT follow-up

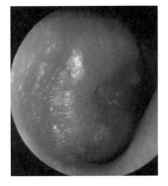 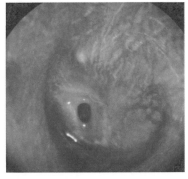

Figure 1.3a &b Bulging tympanic membrane consistent with acute otitis media and ruptured tympanic membrane in AOM.

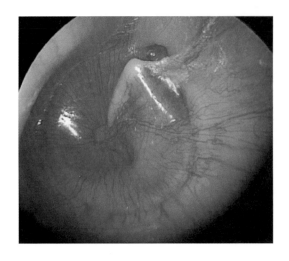

Figure 1.3c Resolving AOM in the left ear without perforation.

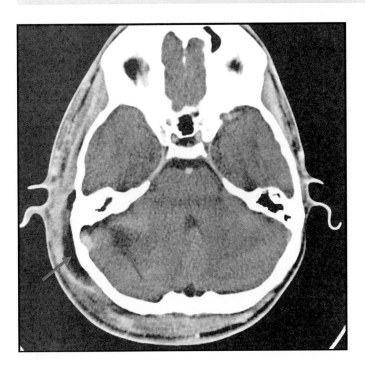

Figure 1.3d Axial CT scan of brain demonstrating rim enhancing hypodensity overlying the right mastoid bone representing a sub-periosteal collection and cerebellar hypodensity suggesting an intra-parenchymal collection. Both resulted from AOM.

1.4 ACUTE MASTOIDITIS

1 History

- Preceding history of acute otitis media (AOM) – pain, hearing loss, otorrhoea
- Typically systemically unwell - those who have received antibiotics may have masked symptoms
- Pain to and behind the ear
- Intracranial symptoms, eg drowsiness, headache, vomiting
- Co-morbidity - immunosuppression
- Previous mastoid surgery

2 Examination

- A subperiosteal mastoid abscess will push the pinna forward giving an asymmetrical appearance when inspected head on
- The post auricular region may have a bulging, fluctuant and tender swelling.
- Otoscopy should show signs of AOM. The posterior bony wall of the ear canal may sag forwards.
- The point of maximal tenderness is typically deep to the cymba concha by pressing through the pinna – this is surface marking of the mastoid antrum.
- Examine for signs of complications i.e. meningism, raised intra-cranial pressure and facial nerve function.

3 Investigation(s)

- FBC, CRP and blood cultures
- The diagnosis of mastoiditis is a clinical one and does not require cross sectional imaging e.g. CT but this may become useful during the patients admission
- When required best initial imaging is contrast enhanced CT of the brain and temporal bones.
- Any patient with an external abscess may also have an intra-cranial complication which initially may be clinically silent.
- If there is a high index of suspicion of an intracranial complication other than meningitis a contrast enhanced MR brain remains the gold standard to exclude pathology.

4 Treatment

- This condition requires admission: IV access and IV antibiotic therapy typically a cephalosporin with good CNS penetration as guided by local hospital protocol.
- Nil by mouth with IV fluids until determined otherwise.
- Senior review <12hours for adults and urgently in children.
- If no improvement or worsening after 24 hours consider cortical mastoidectomy, tissue biopsy of granulations +/- grommet insertion to drain the abscess and ventilate the middle ear
- A drain may be left *in situ* for 24-48 hours

- Continue intravenous antibiotic until apyrexial for 24 hours and then oral antibiotics for one week following discharge.

5 Follow-up and additional information

- Review in one week following discharge
- The absence of a mastoid collection does not exclude mastoiditis
- The absence of AOM or CSOM makes mastoiditis significantly less likely.

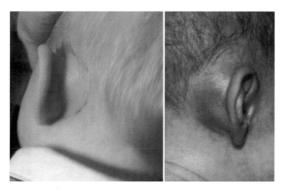

Figures 1.4a & b Early and late acute mastoiditis.

1.5 FACIAL NERVE PALSY (lower motor neurone)

1 History

- Acute onset of unilateral facial weakness
- Otalgia (prodromal pain behind pinna), hyperacusis
- Altered taste
- Otorrhoea – suspect CSOM or the possibility of necrotising otitis externa
- Neurological symptoms especially bulbar symptoms and imbalance (if due to upper motor neurone pathology such as stroke)
- Head injury and skull-base trauma
- Iatrogenic cause – recent otological surgery

2 Examination

- The task is to determine whether the palsy is upper (UMN) or lower motor neurone (LMN) and establish the cause and protect the eye until the weakness resolves.
- Forehead sparing palsies i.e. UMN must be seen urgently by medical registrar as it may reflect a cerebrovascular accident.
- An idiopathic LMN palsy is called a Bell's palsy i.e. diagnosis of exclusion
- Look for vesicles of the ear canal, palate and anterolateral surface of tongue – herpes zoster infection
- Otoscopy – cholesteatoma, haemotympanum, herpes zoster vesicles in EAC, malignant OE

- Tuning fork and free field test of hearing
- Neck - parotid tumours
- Test each branch of VII nerve and grade weakness using the House-Brackmann classification (briefly: grade 1 normal, grade 3 able to close eye, grade 4 unable to close eye, grade 6 complete palsy with no tone in face) (see Table 1.5)
- Associated lower cranial nerve testing – Ramsay Hunt patients can develop bulbar palsy

3 Investigation(s)

- Audiological assessment +/- stapedial reflex testing as outpatient <1/12
- MRI head if suspected posterior fossa lesion i.e. recurrent facial palsy or slow to resolve on follow-up or in child – may be requested in OPD following senior ENT review
- Ophthalmology referral for eye care if incomplete closure at 3/52
- A+E referral to neurosurgery if following head injury with high resolution CT temporal bones and brain.

4 Treatment

- Bell's Palsy/Ramsay-Hunt:
  - oral prednisolone – 50mg OD 10/7 (evidence-based)
  - oral antiviral – acyclovir 800mg five times/day 1/52 (not evidence-based) for

Zoster and Zoster sine herpete infections
- Eye care: viscotears drops QDS, lacrilube BD, eye taped closed at night.

5 Follow-up and additional information

- Bell's palsy/Ramsay Hunt syndrome does not require admission
- Patient should be seen in OPD <2/52 with hearing test on arrival
- Advise that significant recovery occurs over 6 weeks but may take 12 months
- Up to 20% may have incomplete recovery especially if initial total palsy or Ramsay-Hunt
- Document House-Brackmann grade at each visit
- Ophthalmology review if incomplete eye closure at 3/52
- Facial physiotherapy may be helpful if palsy is slow to resolve

Summary of causes of facial nerve palsy:

- Viral (7%), bacterial (4%, dehiscent fallopian canal exposing nerve to toxins), trauma, tumour, central (MS, CVA, Glioma), autoimmune (sarcoid).

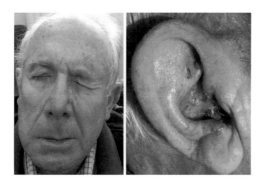

Figure 1.5a&b Right facial nerve palsy with associated with herpetic vesicles on the right ear (Ramsey Hunt syndrome).

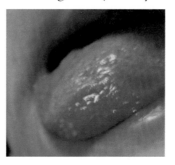

Figure 1.5c Vesicles can occur on any area innervated by nervus intermedius (anterior 2/3 tongue, EAC, pinna, soft palate).

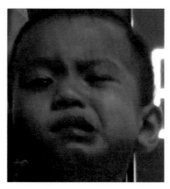

Figure 1.5d A child with a right Bell's palsy.

Table 1.5 House-Brackmann classification of facial nerve paralysis.

Degree of Injury	Grade	Definition
Normal	I	**Normal** – no weakness.
Mild dysfunction (barely noticeable)	II	Slight weakness noticeable only on close inspection. Complete eye closure with minimal effort Slight asymmetry of smile with maximal effort. Synkinesis barely noticeable, contracture, or spasm absent.
Moderate Dysfunction (obvious difference)	III	Obvious weakness, but not disfiguring May not be able to lift eyebrow **Complete eye closure** and strong asymmetrical mouth movement with maximal effort. Obvious but not disfiguring synkinesis, mass movement or spasm.
Moderately severe dysfunction	IV	Obvious disfiguring weakness Inability to lift brow **Incomplete eye closure** and asymmetry of mouth with maximal effort

		Several Synkinesis, mass movement, spasm
Severe dysfunction	V	Motion barely perceptible Incomplete eye closure, slight movement corner mouth Synkinesis, contracture and spasm usually absent
Total Paralysis	VI	**No movement, loss of tone**, no synkinesis, contracture or spasm.

1.6 SUDDEN SENSORI-NEURAL HEARING LOSS (SSNHL)

1 History

- An ENT emergency
- Time of onset – sudden = <3days
- Recent ear surgery or head injury
- Preceding viral infection (mumps, measles, herpes zoster)
- Risk factors similar to cardiac diseases (eg high cholesterol and other lipids, smoking)
- Drug history and FH of ototoxicity (i.e. Gentamicin, Neomycin, Streptomycin, Furosemide, Quinine, Chloroquine and Cisplatin).

2 Examination

- Otoscopy - exclude conductive causes e.g. ear wax impaction, middle ear effusion
- Tuning fork test - should be consistent with SNHL: Rinne's +ve (AC>BC) in affected ear or Rinne false –ve if dead ear (BC>AC), Weber's lateralising to better ear
- Cranial nerve examination looking for nystagmus, facial weakness and cerebellar signs – SSNHL may occasionally represent a focal CVA.

3 Investigation(s)

- Pure tone audiogram to be performed ideally <24hrs - SNHL (no air bone gap). SSNHL defined as deterioration in bone conduction thresholds in 3 contiguous frequencies of 30dBL or greater over a period of less than 3 days.
- All other tests may be performed as outpatient
- Bloods are resource intensive. Discuss with seniors but consider: FBC, ESR, blood glucose, lipid profile, clotting screen, thyroid function tests, viral titres, Lyme serology, serum angiotensin converting enzyme levels, rheumatoid factor, anti-nuclear antibody, cytoplasmic anti-neutrophil cytoplasmic antigen, fluorescent treponemal antibody and OTOblot assay
- CXR - to exclude mediastinal sarcoidosis
- MRI cerebellopontine angle and internal auditory meatus to exclude tumours such as acoustic neuroma (up to 10% associated with sudden SNHL) as an outpatient.

4 Treatment

- Treatment is dependent on local department protocol i.e. inpatient vs outpatient
- Evidence based therapy is oral prednisolone 1mg/kg (up to 60mg od) for 5 days, consider PPI cover. Intra-tympanic steroids may be offered if oral steroids are contraindicated or ineffective.
- Oral antivirals may be offered though without

evidence base - acyclovir 800mg 5 times a day for 7 days or valacyclovir 500mg bd for 7 days
- Admission for Carbogen therapy (5% carbon dioxide, 95% oxygen; 15 minutes every hour for 12hrs) is not evidence based.
- Daily audiograms may help guide treatment.

5 Follow-up and additional information

- Up to 60% of patients will recover hearing spontaneously with no treatment
- If using Carbogen and improvement is seen at 48 hrs then continue treatment. If no improvement: discharge with prednisolone and acyclovir
- Review in 2 weeks with audiology.

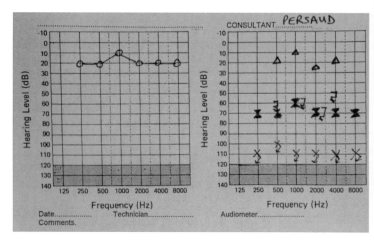

CONSULTANT.... PERSAUD

Figure 1.6a Pure tone audiograms showing profound sensori-neural hearing loss on the left and normal hearing on the right (Δ unmasked bone conduction, O air conduction, shaded X shadow point, arrowed x off scale arrowed] masked left bone conduction off scale).

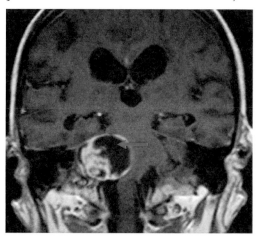

Figure 1.6b A sudden bleed into an acoustic neuroma may result in sudden sensori-neural hearing loss.

1.7 ACUTE VERTIGO

1 History

- Vertigo is an illusory sense of movement often associated with nausea/vomiting.
- General imbalance ('off legs') or pre-syncopal dizziness is admitted under and investigated by general medicine. Ask the patient to commit to which of these descriptors best describes their symptoms.
- Obtain a clear history regarding the mode of onset and associated illness at the time of the primary event.
- Establish the duration of symptoms. Seconds of vertigo suggest benign paroxysmal positional vertigo (BPPV). Hours suggest possible Meniere's disease and days suggests labyrinthitis/vestibular neuronitis.
- Meniere's disease is a diagnosis of exclusion best made in OPD by a senior ENT surgeon and not in primary care. Take care when accepting a label of 'Meniere's disease'.
- A focal CVA or posterior circulation TIA can often mimic 'labyrinthitis'. Take care when accepting an arteriopath with a diagnosis of labyrinthitis.
- Trauma or recent ear surgery
- Also consider central causes such as TIA/CVA, and medical causes such as cardiovascular, endocrine and metabolic especially diabetes

2 Examination

- Full neurological examination, including cranial nerves – to help identify central pathology
- Otoscopy – Otitis media, cholesteatoma
- Nystagmus present – determine what type it is (horizontal, torsional, up/down beating – this suggests CNS pathology), in which direction of gaze it is exacerbated and the direction of the fast corrective saccadic component.
- Pure tone audiology
- Dix – Hallpike Test (see below) – If positive = BPPV
- Romberg and Unterbergers test (see below) are not pathognomonic for labrynthine failure but a negative test makes such a diagnosis less likely.
- Fistula test
- Head impulse

3 Investigation(s)

- Most patients with vertigo will not require admission for investigations – discuss all cases with second on-call if considering to admit under ENT
- Medics should have excluded general or systemic disease e.g. Anaemia, ischaemic heart disease, diabetes mellitus, thyroid dysfunction and CVA
- Outpatient pure tone audiogram (PTA) and MRI of internal auditory meatus to exclude acoustic neuroma if diagnosis unclear
- Vestibular function tests may be required by senior ENT doctor

4 Treatment

- Treatment will depend upon the likely diagnosis which may not be made at primary or secondary presentation.
- Admit only if vertiginous and unable to mobilise or retain fluids and A+E have excluded a central lesion. The gold standard is an MR of brainstem and posterior fossa at 48hrs from symptom onset.
- Supportive therapy eg IV fluids if vomiting and short term vestibular sedation (eg im prochlorperazine)
- Labyrinthitis – vestibular suppressant for acute attack – Prochlorperazine 5mg buccal/12.5mg IM +/- PO Prednisolone if SNHL. In patients who do not compensate – consider vestibular rehabilitation
- BPPV – Epley's Manoeuvre
- Meniere's Disease:
  o Prophylaxis: avoid salt and caffeine, Bendroflumethiazide 2.5mg OD and Betahistine 16mg TDS
  o Acute attacks: Prochlorperazine 5mg buccal

5 Follow-up and additional information

- In about 33% of patients no obvious aetiology is found
- Ask patient to keep daily vertigo record – time and duration of each attack
- Review in one month and if no better refer to specialist balance clinic.

Dix-Hallpike Test

- Sit patient upright on bed, with head turned approximately 30 degrees to one side
- With your hands supporting the patients head on both sides, lower the patient flat onto the bed with the head extending over the side of the bed by approximately 30 degrees
- If positive, after a few seconds the patient will complain of vertigo and a torsional geotropic (clockwise when testing the right ear, and anticlockwise with the left) down beating nystagmus will be present
- Nystagmus lasts for 10-20 seconds and is fatigable on repetition
- Test the other ear by facing the patient to other side whilst sat up
- If the results are incongruent or atypical, consider acoustic neuroma or a central cause and organise an MRI

Romberg's Test

- The patient stands with feet together and hands by their side
- Ask the patient to close their eyes
- Positive if the patient sways/falls
- Stand near the patient and be ready to catch them if they do fall

Unterberger's Test

- Ask the patient to close their eyes
- Hands stretched, palms facing upwards
- March on the spot
- Positive if the patient rotates on the spot, with rotation towards the side of the lesion

Head Impulse Test

- Ensure prior to performing this test that the patient does not suffer from cervical spine disease
- Examine active and passive neck rotation
- Patient to fix gaze at some point behind the examiner
- Gently rotate the head 30degrees from the midline to right and left
- Acutely rotate the head back towards the midline and assess whether the gaze lost fixation which led to a re-fixation saccade; this suggests loss of vestibulo-occular reflex on the side the head was turned towards
- If fixation was maintained this helps exclude a labyrinthine pathology.

1.8 PINNA LACERATION AND HAEMATOMA AURIS

1 History

- Mechanism of injury – dirty
- Age of injury
- Any previous attempts at aspiration/drainage
- Any previous cases of haematoma or chronic pinna deformity
- Recurrent or prolonged cases of pinna haematoma causes necrosis of the pinna cartilage and can result in "cauliflower ear" deformity
- Remember to exclude any head injury as a result of trauma.

2 Examination

- Advanced trauma life support (ATLS) assessment of trauma guided by mechanism of injury
- Assess for haematoma (fluctuant or tense) or ecchymosis (mildly swollen and discoloured without loss of shape) and laceration.
- Otoscopy – injury to the ear canal, TM perforation and haemotympanum, cerebrospinal fluid (CSF) otorrhoea (water like discharge from ear).

3 Investigation(s)

- If any sign of trauma to base of skull such as bruising to mastoid (Battle's sign) or haemotympanum – for A+E to formally exclude traumatic brain injury by CT head.

4 Treatment

- Thoroughly clean pinna – often only possible following the infiltration of local anaesthesia ideally with a dental syringe, needle and Lignospan (Lidocaine HCL 2% and epinephrine 1:80,000)
- Assess for tissue loss and if possible close in layers with 3.0 vicryl to cartilage and 5.0 prolene to skin.
- A pinna which is held with any tissue bridge still takes remarkably well.
- Discuss with seniors before attempting to reattach a completely avulsed pinna especially if bitten.
- Incise and drain pinna haematoma under LA or GA and aseptic conditions. Aspiration may help with diagnosis but will often lead to reaccumulation.
- Pressure needs to be applied to the pinna to prevent reaccumulation. Use silastic sheets or dental rolls sutured on both sides of the pinna with through and through mattress non-absorbable sutures
- A corrugated drain is sometimes left *in situ* (Figure 1.8b) for 24 hours
- Alternatively, saline or betadine soaked cotton wool can be moulded to the contour of the pinna and applied with an overlying pressure hand bandage
- Provide prophylactic antibiotics and consider

tetanus booster if required.

5 Follow-up and additional information

- Review patient in 3-4 days
- If the haematoma has reaccumulated, repeat incision and drainage may be required
- Re-review the patient until satisfied that no haemtoma is present and the wound has healed
- Remove dental rolls, silastic sheet, drain
- Monitor for cauliflower ear caused by infection between the cartilage and perichondrium.

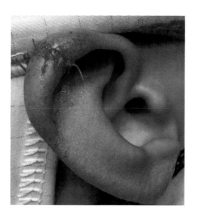

Figure 1.8a Pinna laceration from a dog bite.

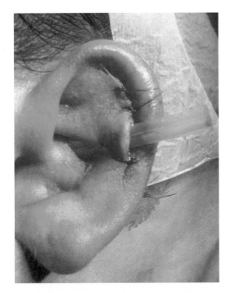

Figure 1.8b Incision and drainage of a pinna haematoma.

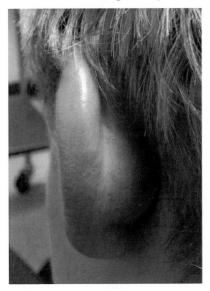

Figure 1.8c Posterior pinna haematoma.

1.9 TEMPORAL BONE FRACTURE (inc CSF LEAK)

1 History

- Associated with significant head and brain injury.
- Patients should never be admitted under ENT unless a traumatic brain injury is excluded by neurosurgeons. Note: a 'normal CT brain' on arrival does not exclude cerebral contusion / injury.
- Ask about mechanism of head injury (high impact energy required to fracture the temporal bone, lateral force over mastoid leads to longitudinal fracture which is 80% of all temporal bone fracture)
- Watery discharge (CSF) from nose and/or ear
- Vertigo
- Hearing loss
- Facial weakness – must ask referring clinician to grade facial nerve function using the House-Brackmann system and determine whether the weakness occurred immediately after injury or if was delayed.
- Other associated injuries.

2 Examination

- A+E & neurosurgeons to stabilise the patient using ATLS protocols.
- Bedside otological examination. Look for nystagmus on looking away from affected ear, CSF

otorrhoea, drum perforation and facial nerve palsy.

- Facial nerve palsy (immediate complete, immediate incomplete or delayed) (House-Brackmann grading)
- Tuning fork hearing tests.

3 Investigation(s)

- High resolution CT temporal bone only if reparative or decompressive surgery needed i.e. refractory CSF otorrhoea or immediate total facial palsy
- Pure tone audiogram when patient is stable
- Beta-2 transferrin test to confirm CSF otorrhoea/rhinorrhoea – there is no other way to confirm or exclude a CSF leak.

4 Treatment

- External ear canal laceration, haemotympanum or ruptured TM:
  - o Conservative, avoid straining.
- Nystagmus and nausea/vomiting:
  - o PRN Stemetil and vestibular rehabilitation exercises
  - o Usually resolves completely after 3-6months
- CN7 palsy:
  - o Immediate complete palsy: discuss with neuro-otologist regarding

exploration/decompression/repair of facial nerve
- o Immediate incomplete: suggest a functional non-severed nerve, recovers with time.
- o Delayed palsy – give 10 days oral steroid if not contraindicated
- CSF leak:
  - o Conservative with bed rest, head elevation and stool softeners
  - o No sneezing, no coughing, no straining, no nose blowing
  - o Usually closes by 1 week
  - o If leak persists: referral to neuro-otologist
  - o Consider lumbar drain
  - o Antibiotics controversial, risk of meningitis is approximately 15% (*haemophilus and streptococcus*)
- Hearing loss, consider:
  - o Tympanoplasty or ossiculoplasty for conductive hearing loss (surgical exploration after 2 months if hearing loss is >30dB, unless only hearing ear.
  - o Contra-lateral routing of sound (CROS) aid or Bone conduction hearing aid (BCHA) for single sided deafness.

5 Follow-up and additional information

- Temporal bone fracture should never be admitted under care of ENT given need for A+E to manage co-existing traumatic brain injury.
- 8 weeks for pure tone audiogram and water precautions until OPD review

- Longitudinal fractures are longitudinal to the long axis of the petrous portion of the temporal bone. Often runs through the middle ear and ear canal leading to conductive hearing loss and haematorrohea.
- Transverse fractures run across the long axis of the petrous temporal bone and are more likely to run through the otic capsule and cause CSF leak, facial palsy and total nerve hearing loss (dead ear).

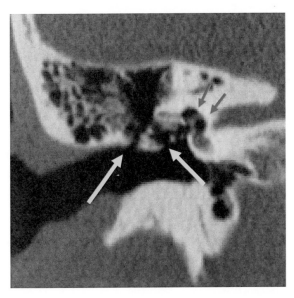

Figure 1.9 Coronal CT image showing fractures (yellow arrows) of the temporal bone as well as a pneumolabyrinth (red arrows) (this patient will therefore have profound SNHL).

1.10 INFECTED PREAURICULAR SINUS

1 History

- Congenital pit anterior to root of the helix of ear
- Intermittent discharge from pit
- Ask about mucoid discharge from neck and hearing loss or renal dysfunction (may suggest brachio-oto-renal syndrome).

2 Examination

- Examine for bilateral pits
- Look for signs of infection or abscess formation
- Inspect neck for small sinus with mucoid discharge [brachio-oto-renal (BOR) syndrome].

3 Investigation(s)

- FBC if infection present
- Audiogram and tympanogram
- Patient with neck cysts/sinus and FH may benefit from renal ultrasound scan as outpatient.

4 Treatment

- Analgesia
- Antibiotics (oral or intravenous) depending on the severity of infection
- Elective surgical excision to remove entire tract surrounding soft tissue as well as any cartilage involved when not actively infected.

5 Follow-up and additional information

- After surgical excision to ensure no residual discharging site.

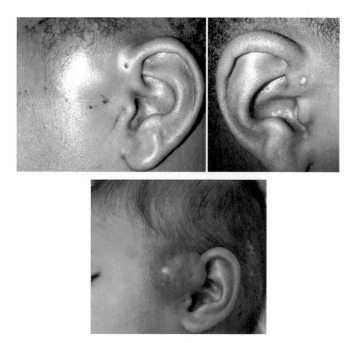

Figures 1.10a-c Infected preauricular sinus with and without surrounding cellulitis/collection.

1.11 PERICHONDRITIS OF THE EXTERNAL EAR

1 History

- History of some form of trauma such as a high ear piercing through cartilage, insect bite, laceration, chemical injury, frostbite etc
- Skin infection (erysipelas) may spread to the perichondrial layer (perichondritis) or cartilage (chondritis).

2 Examination

- Classical signs of inflammation: redness, painful, swollen and hot.
- May develop into a subperichondrial abscess
- Usually localised condition, although strep septicaemia is possible
- If recurrent consider relapsing polychondritis

3 Investigation(s)

- FBC
- Microscopy culture and sensitivity (MC&S) of any pus present
- Consider biopsy is actively considering relapsing polychondritis

4 Treatment

- Local and intravenous broad spectrum antibiotics that covers both gram negative and positive organisms
- Incise and drain subperichondrial abscess if present
- May required debridement of necrotic cartilage

5 Follow-up and additional information

- OPD 1/52 to ensure resolution of infection and sensitivities of microbiological specimens

1.12 RELAPSING POLYCHONDRITIS

1 History

- Chronic inflammatory condition affecting cartilage in the pinna, nose and laryngo-trachea
- Characterised by acute exacerbations and remissions.

2 Examination

- Fever in acute phase
- Affects pinna, nasal septum (saddling and collumela retraction), larynx and eyes (conjunctivitis, keratitis, uveitis).

3 Investigation(s)

- Raised inflammatory markers – none are diagnostic
- Clinical diagnosis supported by histology
- Audiogram – may be associated with auto-immune hearing loss

4 Treatment

- Liaise with rheumatologist on call
- High dose steroids to induce remission (30-60mg/day)
- Low dose steroids to suppress recurrence (5-10mg/day)
- Immunosuppressants: azathioprine or methotrexate
- Anti-CD4 monoclonal antibody and minocycline

5 Follow-up and additional information

- By the multi-professional team including laryngologist and rheumatologist.

1.13 FURUNCULOSIS

1 History

- Exquisite otalgia from an infected hair follicle located in the outer third of the ear canal
- Often difficult to distinguish between furunculosis and severe diffuse otitis externa
- Serosanguinous discharge
- Little or no hearing loss.

2 Examination

- Well circumscribed deep skin infection
- Oedema, cellulitis and inflammation confined to the lateral third of the canal
- Deep canal and tympanic membrane appear normal.

3 Investigation(s)

- MC&S (*staph aureus* is commonest causative organism)

4 Treatment

- Analgesia
- Abscess will eventually rupture if allowed to follow a natural course
- Incision and drainage can speed up the process
- Oral or intravenous antibiotics
- Topical aluminium acetate solution is an astringent and hygroscopic agent.

5 Follow-up and additional information

- In recurrent cases consider 14 days of flucloxacillin and eradication therapy with nasal mupirocin
- Bacterial interference therapy ie implanting a non-pathogenic *staph aureus* (strain 502A) to recolonise nose and skin.

1.14 TRAUMATIC PERFORATION OF THE TYMPANIC MEMBRANE (inc NAI)

1 History

- Barotrauma including blow to head, blast injury, diving
- Syringing ear
- History of previous perforation or chronic ear discharge (may suggest chronic perforation)
- Be suspicious of non –accidental injury (NAI), especially if a child with incompatible history, delay in presentation, inappropriate affect.

2 Examination

- Blood in canal
- Perforated tympanic membrane
- Hearing loss/tinnitus
- Pinna trauma and sign of brain injury
- Bruising on body.

3 Investigation(s)

- Consider audiological assessment.

4 Treatment

- Water precautions i.e. no swimming and cotton wool + Vaseline to conchal bowl if in shower
- Routine antibiotic prophylaxis is not required
- Must discuss with senior on-call and refer to child safeguarding team via paediatric registrar if suspicious of non-accidental injury

5 Follow-up and additional information

- 6 weeks for repeat audiological assessment and water precautions until review.

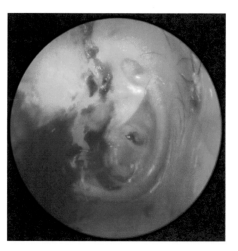

Figure 1.14a Clinical photograph showing blood in the deep ear canal of a child and a small traumatic anterior perforation.

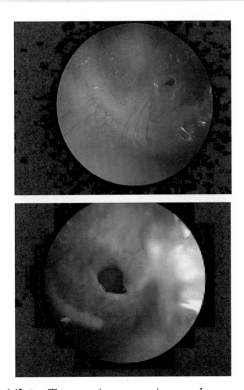

Figure 1.14b&c Traumatic tympanic membrane perforation, classically small, jagged edges, occasionally triangular shaped.

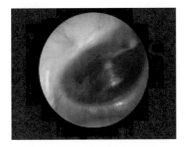

Figure 1.14d Traumatic haematympanum.

1.15 NECROTISING OTITIS EXTERNA (NOE)

1 History

- Prolonged otitis externa with intense pain out of proportion to signs
- Elderly, diabetic, renal disease, immunocompromised
- Facial nerve palsy
- Systemic illness

2 Examination

- Oto-microscopy – suction, swab and biopsy for histology and microbiology
- Facial nerve palsy (House-Brackmann grading)
- Other cranial nerve palsy.

3 Investigation(s)

- FBC, blood culture
- Microbiology swab from ear discharge
- Biopsy abnormal looking tissue if concerned about a neoplastic process
- High resolution CT temporal bone looking for bony erosion or skull base involvement
- HBA1C can delineate poor diabetic control.

4 Treatment

- Multidisciplinary management with microbiology, radiology and skull-base ENT surgeon
- Admit for IV antibiotics with good bony penetrance and *Pseudomonas sp* and G-ve cover under the guidance of microbiology.
- Often require 6/52 if IV therapy and 4/12 of oral therapy.
- Analgesia.
- Regular meticulous microsuction and topical antibiotic and steroid therapy
- Surgical debridement of necrotic bone is infrequently required.
- Correct underlying medical problems (for example neutropenia, uncontrolled diabetes)
- Reassessment of facial nerve palsy
- Eye protection if required.

5 Follow-up and additional information

- Weekly review following discharge to monitor progress and supervise course of protracted oral antibiotics
- A high level of suspicion is required for prompt diagnosis and treatment to avoid complications such as cranial nerve involvement.
- It is associated with a mortality of up to 50%.

Chapter 2

Nose

2.1 FOREIGN BODY IN THE NOSE (inc RHINOLITH)

1 History

- History typically from witness or adult with strong suspicion
- Nature of foreign body (organic or non-organic)
- Duration of insertion.
- Chronic FB results in unilateral foul smelling nasal discharge
- A rhinolith may be an incidental finding in an adult.

2 Examination

- Anterior rhinoscopy usually shows FB lodged between the septum and anterior end of the inferior turbinate
- Vestibulitis from chronic rhinorrhoea if FB present for some time
- Reduced nasal airflow on misting test with a cold lack spatula

3 Investigation(s)

- X-ray is NOT effective at excluding a FB. Be led by parental history.

4 Treatment

- Always perform with nursing assistance and never fight an uncooperative child.
- The first attempt at FB removal is the best - do NOT 'have a go' if you are not trained are liable to render the child uncooperative for further attempts and thus committed to a examination under anaesthesia (EUA).
- Do aim to remove the FB on the day of referral - it is NOT appropriate to refer such patients to an outpatient clinic.
- Child and parental cooperation is key. Spend time to win the trust of both. Allow the child to handle the instruments and headlight. Approach in a non-threatening manner. Decongestion and soft suction catheters may improve visualisation
- Explain the process to parents and gain consent.
- With child on parents lap inspect the nose with an otoscope.
- Anterior spherical FB may be removed by placing a Jobson Horne probe above and beyond the FB and pulling the FB out by sweeping the instrument gently forward pivoting at the upper alar rim. If fabric or paper a small crocodile forceps is effective. Parents may need to hold the child's arms for reassurance.

- Button batteries must be removed as soon as possible (ideally within 2 hours).
- A rhinolith should be removed under GA to avoid pain, ensure complete removal and irrigation.

5 Follow-up and additional information

- If confident that FB is removed – none required.
- If suspicion of retained FB discuss with senior re: need to EUA if possible aspiration risk. Alternatively follow-up closely in OPD.
- Foul smelling unilateral nasal discharge may represent a retained FB – parents should be aware of need for re-examination in such circumstance.
- A rhinolith is a nasal concretion originating from a small inorganic FB on which calcium, magnesium carbonate and phosphates are deposited over many years.

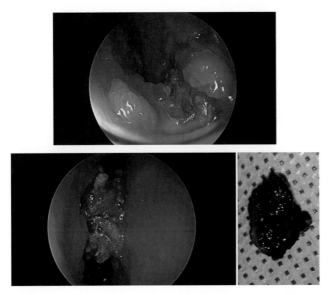

Figures 2.1a-c A rhinolith in the nose of an adult who was referred for nasal obstruction (a rhinolith *in situ*, b rhinolith mobilised, c rhinolith specimen).

2.2 FOREIGN BODY IN THE BRONCHUS (inc Speaking Valve)

1 History

- Witnessed FB ingestion/inhalation (cough, choking and dyspnoea at the time of event is the most sensitive indicator for airway FB)
- Wheezing
- 'Asthma' unresponsive to bronchodilators
- Blood stain sputum and chronic cough with treatment refractory chest infection
- Laryngectomy patient may report speaking valve missing.

2 Examination

- Child may be wholly asymptomatic
- Monophonic wheezing in previously well child
- Difficulty breathing
- Poor air entry on one side
- Intercostal recession and flaring of nostril.

3 Investigation(s)

- CXR (may be normal or hyperinflated if FB is having a ball valve effect).

4 Treatment

- EUA is the only way to exclude FB and must be performed urgently.
- Rigid bronchoscopy and retrieval of FB using optical forceps under general anaesthesia
- May require assistance from respiratory colleagues for bronchoscopy or thoracic team for possible thoracotomy
- Speaking valve lodged in the bronchus may be fished out with forceps taped to flexible nasendoscope (see Figures 2.2f&g) without the need for a GA.

5 Follow-up and additional information

- To confirm resolution of symptoms

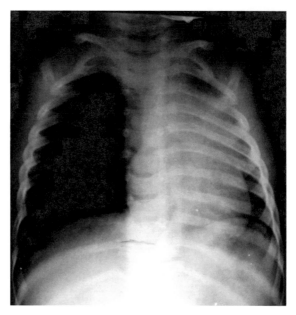

Figure 2.2a Chest x-ray showing hyperflation of the right lung with mediastinal shift to the left as a result of a FB in the right main bronchus having a ball valving effect.

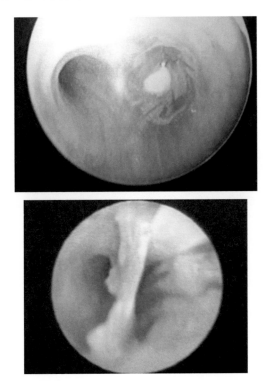

Figure 2. 2b&c Foreign bodies in the right main bronchus (peanut and apple).

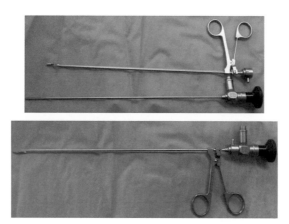

Figure 2.2d&e Optical forceps and endoscopy for retrieval of foreign body in the lungs (before and after assembling).

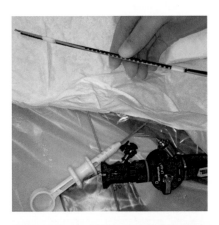

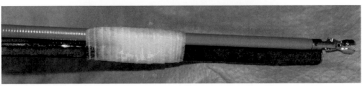

Figure 2.2f&g Nasendoscope taped to OGD biopsy forceps for retrieval of speaking valve from bronchus in a laryngectomy patient.

2.3 EPISTAXIS ANTERIOR

1 History

- Initial side of bleeding ie left or right
- Frequency or bleeds and duration of episode
- Attempt to control bleed with digital compression
- Risk factor assessment - trauma including digital and surgery, DH incl. aspirin and warfarin.

2 Examination

- Assess amount of blood loss and decide if resuscitation is necessary
- With head light, suction and assistant decongest the nose with cotton wool soaked in vasoconstrictor
- Examine Little's area (commonest site of bleeding) and identify the bleeding point(s).

3 Investigation(s)

- FBC, clotting and G+S, if indicated.

4 Treatment

- Airway, breathing and circulation treatment and resuscitate as necessary
- Lean forward (Trotter's position) - avoid swallowing blood
- Pinch soft lower 1/3 of nose, NOT the bony bridge, for 10 minutes
- Icepack on nasal bridge or forehead
- ENT referral if bleeding has not ceased in 20 minutes
- Cauterise bleeding point with silver nitrate after numbing the area with co-phenylcaine on a ribbon gauze for at least 5 minutes
- Repeat cauterization if necessary
- Naseptin cream or Bactraban ointment (if patient is allergic to peanuts) should be applied to cauterised area twice a day for 1 week
- Advise patient not to eat or drink for next hour due to use of local anaesthetic which may be affect throat
- In the majority of anterior epistaxis the above works and the patient can be discharged. Rarely one would need to insert a nasal pack such as merocel and observe for 24 hours. Insert pack horizontally i.e. parallel to nasal floor.

5 Follow-up and additional information

- Check for septal perforation following cauterisation
- Advise patient not to place finger in nose post cautery. Dab any liquid leaking from nose with

> damp cloth – fluid is caustic.
> - If nasal packing is used for more than 24 hours, a broad spectrum antibiotic (eg co-amoxiclav) should be given to prevent toxic shock syndrome.

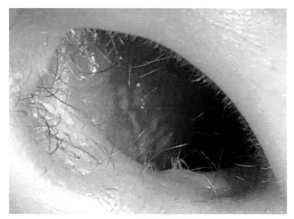

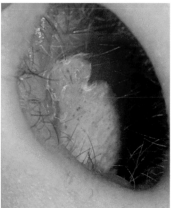

Figures 2.3a & b Little's area on the right septum before and after cauterisation with silver nitrate.

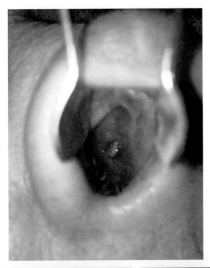

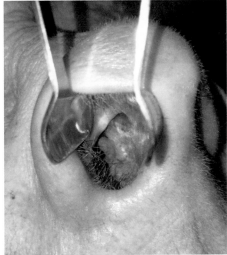

Figures 2.3c & d Bleeding vessel in Little's area on the right septum before and after cauterisation with silver nitrate (Cophenylcaine was used as topical anaesthesia).

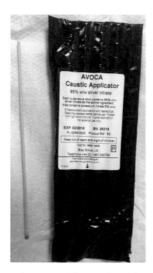

Figure 2.3e Silver nitrate sticks and packet material.

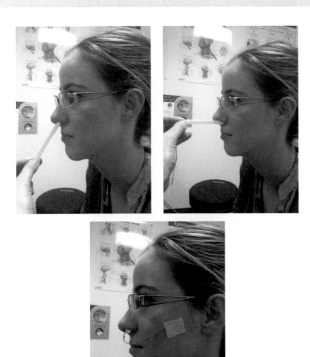

Figure 2.3f & g Incorrect and correct way of inserting a merocel nasal pack for epistaxis management, only if it is impossible to control bleeding with cauterisation.

2.4 EPISTAXIS POSTERIOR

1 History

- As per anterior epistaxis
- Elderly patient
- Patient typically describes blooding running into back of throat. If no bleeding point is seen anteriorly and blood seen trickling down the back of oropharynx, this would suggest posterior bleed. To confirm a posterior bleeding point, perform flexible naso-pharyngo-laryngoscopy (FNE) or rigid nasendoscopy.

2 Examination

- As per anterior epistaxis
- Anterior rhinoscopy to inspect Little's area
- Rigid endoscope (preferably) or FNE to identify posterior bleeding area
- Usually Woodruff plexus on the lateral nasal wall behind the posterior end of the inferior turbinate.

3 Investigation(s)

- FBC
- Clotting
- G&S.

4 Treatment

- Posterior and anterior packs
- Specially designed posterior packs include the Brighton balloon and posterior length Rapid Rhino. If these are unavailable, a Foley catheter inflated in the post nasal space with gentle anterior traction maintained by umbilical cord clamp to anterior nares wrapped in gauze to prevent tissue necrosis. BIPP dressing packed anterior to balloon.
- If patient is still bleeding after 48 hours of packing consider sphenopalatine artery ligation or embolisation of the terminal branches of internal maxillary artery (IMAX).

5 Follow-up and additional information

- To check for adhesions
- Rigid endoscope is ideal to examine nose because of better optics and one hand is free for suctioning and cauterisation.

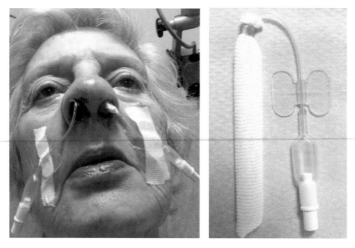

Figure 2.4a & b Rapid rhino balloon tampon for epistaxis after and before insertion.

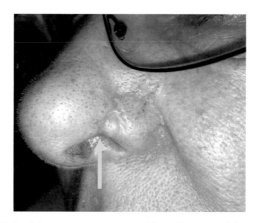

Figure 2.4c Alar notching caused by clip on a foley catheter used for posterior epistaxis control.

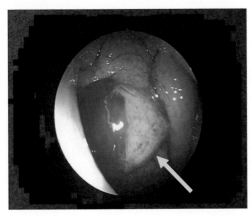

Figure 2.4d Posterior epistaxis caused by a post-nasal mass.

2.5 EPISTAXIS IN SPECIAL CONDITIONS

1 History

- Young or old patient
- Anticoagulant therapy eg warfarin
- Alcoholic (B12 and folate acid deficiency leading to thrombocytopenia).

2 Examination

- Bruising on body
- Telangectasia present (Hereditory Haemorrhagic Telangectasia (HHT))
- Nasal lesion present (eg pyogenic granuloma, juvenile angiofibroma in male teenagers).

3 Investigation(s)

- FBC, Coagulation screen, G&S.

4 Treatment

- **High INR**: consider prothrombin complex concentrate (PCC), which is a combination of

clotting factors II, VII, IX and X as well as protein C and S (trade name Beriplex, Octoplex or Kcnetra)
- **Pyogenic granuloma**: surgical excision
- **Juvenile angiofibroma**: Nasal packing and embolisation of internal maxillary artery followed by surgical excision and drilling out the basisphenoid region via a mid-facial degloving approach
- **HHT**: Kaltostat or other dissolvable nasal pack soaked in adrenaline; tranexamic acid.

5 Follow-up and additional information

- Yes, duration depends on cause identified

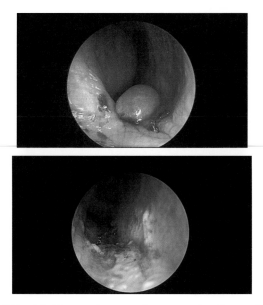

Figure 2.5a &b Pyogenic granuloma on the floor of nose causing intermittent epistaxis before and after removal.

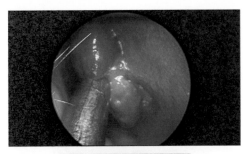

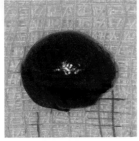

Figure 2.5c & d Pyogenic granuloma on the nasal septum *in situ* and specimen.

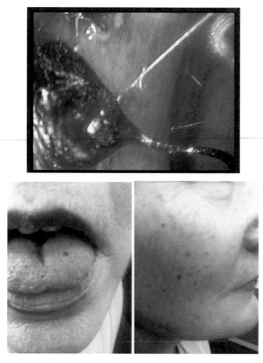

Figure 2.5e-f Hereditary haemorrhagic telangestasia affecting the nose, lips and face.

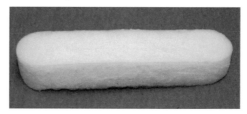

Figure 2.5g Dissolvable nasopore for acute epistaxis in HHT patients.

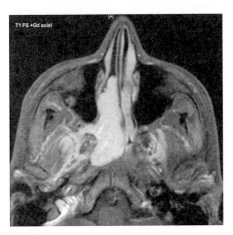

Figure 2.5h MRI showing a high signal lesion consistent with a juvenile angiofibroma.

2.6 FRACTURED NOSE

1 History

- Mechanism of injury
- Low or high impact injury
- Any other associated injuries
- Loss of consciousness, amnesia, neurological deficit, double vision
- Patient perception of change in shape of nose and history of prior injury and nasal obstruction.

2 Examination

- ABC as per APLS
- Exclude signs of significant head injury requiring A+E neuro-observation (low GCS or significant mechanism of injury or CSF leak) and associated maxilla-facial (bony tenderness and dental malocclusion) and ophthalmological trauma (diplopia and enophthalmos)
- Q1. External nasal deviation?
- Q2. Nasal obstruction?
- Q3. Septal haematoma?
- Q4. Epistaxis?

3 Investigation(s)

- No need for nasal x-ray – only plain films for exclusion of maxillofacial fracture
- CT scan should be requested by referring specialty if skull base fracture suspected.

4 Treatment

- Resuscitate according to ATLS protocol and control any haemorrhage.
- Firm pressure and head flexed with IV access. Occasionally require nasal packing or manipulation of fracture in A+E to allow packing.
- Anterior ethmoidal artery laceration is uncommon but may require control in theatre.
- If haematoma – must admit for urgent drainage.
- If new deformity or obstruction – OPD review in 5/7 with manipulation under anaesthesia (MUA) of fractured nose under LA or GA within first 2 weeks after swelling has subsided.
- Reassure and discharge if no obvious deviation and no functional problem
- Minor open nasal fracture can be reduced under LA, cleaned thoroughly with antiseptic agent and the skin sutured
- Major open nasal fracture may require a GA for reduction and delayed closure of the skin as infection may occur with primary closure.

5 Follow-up and additional information

- If no change to nasal shape or nasal airflow and no haematoma – nil action or follow-up.
- A nose can be fractured without deviation or obstruction, however this will not require treatment
- Plain radiographs are not performed.
- Beware the patient with pre-existing nasal deformity.

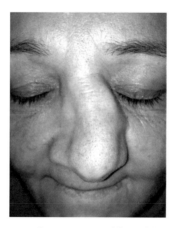

Figure 2.6a Fractured nose caused by a blow from the right side of the face.

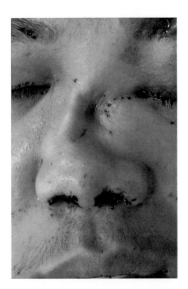

Figure 2.6b Comminuted fracture of the nose (impact from the left side).

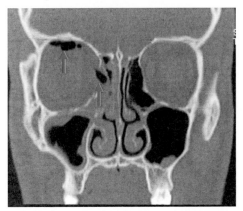

Figure 2.6c Right orbital emphysema resulting from a head trauma (note that this can lead to an acute compartment syndrome with compressive or ischaemic optic nerve neuropathy and blindness).

2.7 SEPTAL HAEMATOMA

1 History

- Usually caused by trauma or iatrogenic e.g. post septoplasty
- Severe pain
- Total or near total nasal obstruction.

2 Examination

- Bulbous, fluctuant, red swelling in anterior septum ("cherry in nose" see Figure 2.3a-c)
- Boggy on palpation with Jobson-Horne probe
- Usually bilateral but can be unilateral.

3 Investigation(s)

- Take bloods for FBC, coagulation screen
- Take swab of any pus or discharge present.

4 Treatment

- List for GA drainage as an emergency.
- Horizontal incision at inferior limit of collection,

washout and small drain inserted if pus drained.
- Quilt septal mucosa to septal cartilage with 4.0 vicryl and pack both nasal passages for 48hours with antibiotic soaked ribbon gauze.
- 24hours of IV antibiotic therapy is a minimum.
- 5/7 oral antibiotics

5 Follow-up and additional information

- 5/7 OPD after successful treatment.
- Assess septum for re-accumulation.
- Inform patient of risk of late perforation or saddle nose deformity

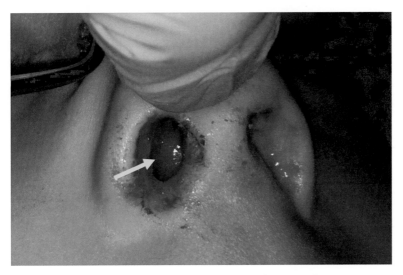

Figure 2.7a Unilateral septal haematoma (cherry red septum).

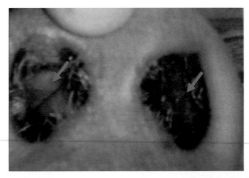

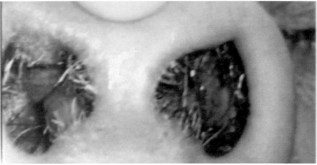

Figure 2.7b &c Bilateral septal haematoma (same patient with different lighting).

2.8 ACUTE RHINOSINUSITIS (ARS)

1 History

- Nasal obstuction, nasal discharge (anterior or posterior), facial pain/pressure, loss of sense of smell (conductive anosmia)
- Preceding coryzal symptoms
- Fever
- Dental problems, especially if there is swelling of the cheek.

2 Examination

- Rigid nasendoscopy to check for mucopus from sinus openings and the presence of any lesions eg polyps
- Eye examination: visual acuity, pupillary reflex, colour vision (loss of red colour vision is early sign of optic nerve compression)
- Full central and peripheral neurological examination if intracranial complications suspected
- Facial swelling is usually caused by dental abscess rather than sinus disease, therefore inspect the teeth and alveolar margins
- Seek dental input if appropriate.

3 Investigation(s)

- Blood tests, blood culture only if severely ill or complications.
- Microscopy and culture of mucopus from nasal cavity
- Imaging is not required in uncomplicated acute sinusitis unless signs of complications such as periorbital cellulitis and/or suspicion of intracranial abscess.

4 Treatment

- Outpatient management is typical.
- If symptoms <10/7 and not grossly unwell or with signs of complications / immunodeficiency then supportive care only
- Analgesia
- If prolonged symptoms >10/7 and suspicion of acute bacterial sinusitis, antibiotics as per trust policy to cover *streptococcus pneumoniae* and *haemophilus influenzae*. Co-amoxiclav for 1 week is a common first line option with nasal decongestants (otrivine 2-3 drops TDS for no longer than 5 days) and nasal steroid drops for 1/52, steam inhalation and saline douching
- Occasionally antral washout is necessary.

5 Follow-up and additional information

- Uncomplicated cases do not require follow up.
- Persistence of symptoms >3months suggests chronic rhinosinusitis.
- Complications of ARS include: periorbital cellulitis, subperiosteal abscess, Pott's puffy tumour, osteomyelitis, intracranial abscess/subdural empyema and meningitis.

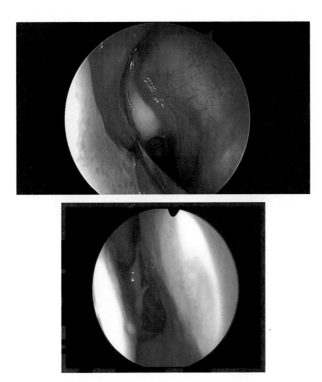

Figure 2.8 Acute rhinosinusitis with pus arising from the left maxillary sinus.

2.9 PERIORBITAL CELLULITIS

1 History

- Preceding URTI and symptoms of acute sinusitis
- Periorbital swelling and pain
- Difficulty eye opening
- Impaired vision

2 Examination

- Demands early joint assessment with ophthalmologists.
- Establish whether the infection is anterior or posterior to the septum which inserts into the orbital rim and tarsal plates.
- Pre-septal infection may progress to post-septal and post-septal infection can be sight and life threatening.
- Examine for active and passive eye opening.
- Red flags for post-septal infection include - proptosis, painful and restricted eye movement
- Reduced acuity begins with impaired colour vision and red desaturation as assessed by Ishihara plates.
- Nasal examination for sinusitis – note that peri-orbital sinusitis can occur without signs of sinusitis.
- GCS – may be complicated by brain abscess
- Cranial nerve examination – may reveal cavernous sinus thrombosis
- Forehead swelling – Pott's puffy tumour.

3 Investigation(s)

- Rhinoscopy to look for signs of acute bacterial sinusitis
- Swab any nasal discharge/pus
- CT head, para-nasal sinus and orbits with contrast and coronal reformatting – if signs of post-septal disease or unable to make assessment or no response to IV therapy.
- Disease is staged by the Chandler classification.

4 Treatment

- Nasal decongestion and steroids and douching
- IV antibiotics guided by local protocol, blood cultures if pyrexial
- Initially half hourly eye observations and 4 hourly neurological observations
- Surgery performed urgently if evidence of reduced visual acuity or an abscess is demonstrated. If surgery not possible and vision is impaired a lateral canthotomy and cantholysis may help decompress the eye.
- Sinus washout may be performed.

5 Follow-up and additional information

- This disease usually complicates acute sinusitis but follow-up is required to ensure the resolution of nasal signs and symptoms. Late recurrence and complications may occur.

- Loss of colour vision is first to go and may be reversible with prompt decompression of eye by drainage of abscess or pressure release by lateral canthotomy.

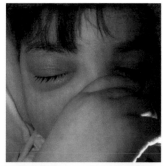

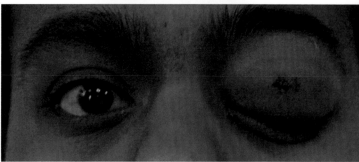

Figure 2.9a&b Periorbital cellulitis.

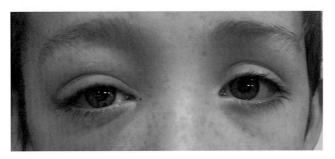

Figure 2.9c Preseptal cellulitis.

2.10 POTT'S PUFFY TUMOUR

1 History

- Headache, fever and tender/fluctuant swelling over forehead
- History of sinusitis or trauma to head
- May be associated with chronic rhinosinusitis or complications of acute rhino-sinusitis
- Most common in adolescents.

2 Examination

- Swinging pyrexia
- Tender fluctuant swelling over frontal region.
- Nasal discharge, congestion, polyposis
- Focal neurological symptoms/reduced GCS/raised intracranial pressure secondary to subdural empyema/abscess.

3 Investigation(s)

- Bloods including culture
- Contrast CT head and para-nasal sinuses and MRI with contrast brain.
- Pus for MC+S.

4 Treatment

- Prolonged course of IV antibiotics typically for 6 weeks followed by oral step down.
- Surgical drainage of pus (via external incision and/or functional endoscopic sinus surgery (FESS)).
- Direct incision may lead to fistulation and frontal sinus surgery may be hazardous.
- Frontal sinus trephine may represent an effective compromise.
- Bony sequestra occasionally require open debridement.
- When there are co-existing intracranial complications (30% of cases) treatment is best decided by a multi-professional team involving surgeons, radiologist and microbiologist.

5 Follow-up and additional information

- Facial scarring or persistent fistula may be a long term sequelae
- Potts Puffy tumour is a subperiosteal collection of an osteomyelitic anterior table of the frontal sinus.
- This condition is associated with intracranial complications in 30% of cases and demands an MR brain with contrast enhancement and repeat assessment as symptoms dictate.
- IV antibiotic treatment should have good bone penetrance and duration commensurate with treating an osteomyelitic process.

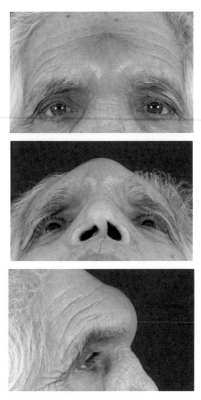

Figures 2.10 a-c Pott's puffy tumour.

2.11 CSF RHINORHOEA

1 History

- Head trauma
- Nasal surgery
- Signs or symptoms of meningism
- If patient obese consider benign intracranial hypertension without hydrocephalus.

2 Examination

- Observe leak with head in dependent position
- Collect sample of fluid for beta-2 transferrin analysis and serum sample for the same.

3 Investigation(s)

- Beta 2 transferin or Tau protein analysis of >0.5ml of fluid to confirm diagnosis; if positive and atraumatic - localise source of leak by CT of skull-base to include temporal bone.
- Fluid glucose testing or 'halo sign' on blotting paper is neither sensitive nor specific for CSF.
- T2 weighted MRI (CSF signal is high)
- High resolution CT scan of skull-base
- Pre-operative intrathecal fluorosceine may be used to further localise.

4 Treatment

- Seek medical attention if signs of meningeal irritation.
- If following head injury – head up bed rest, laxatives for 1/52 surgery and lumbar drain if not settling
- If atraumatic then surgical repair following localisation by endoscopic or open technique with neurosurgeon.

5 Follow-up and additional information

- Yes to ensure no further CSF leak
- A syndrome of raised intracranial pressure (ICP) in the absence of hydrocephalus most often seen in the obese. Chronic raised ICP is suspected to lead to skull base remodelling which predisposes to CSF leak. May also lead to optic nerve atrophy.
- Diagnosis is based on history, slit ventricles on CT and raised ICP on lumbar puncture (LP)
- May require temporary lumbar drain post-op to reduce risk of leak repair failure.

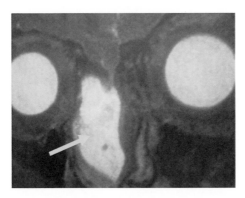

Figure 2.11a T2 weighted MRI showing high signal material in the nose consistent with CSF (note that water is bright on T2 weighted images but dark on T1 weighted images, hence why contrast is never given with T2 weighted MRI).

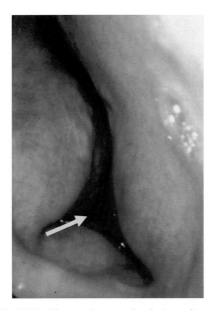

Figure 2.11b CSF Rhinorrhoea which is indistinguishable from allergic rhinorrhoea.

2.12 MUCORMYCOSIS

1 History

- Pyrexia
- Nasal discharge (purulent, black)
- Unilateral headache, facial swelling and pain
- Sinusitis not improving with antibiotic therapy
- Immunocompromised (cancer, transplant, uncontrolled diabetes), skin trauma
- Fungal infection in other areas: lungs (cough), skin (ulcer, blister, erythema), GI tract (nausea and vomiting, abdominal pain), disseminated infection.

2 Examination

- Black nasal discharge with crusting
- Sinuses for signs of infection
- Necrotic black eschars on hard palate and turbinates,
- Proptosis, diplopia, vision loss – early joint assessment with ophthalmology
- Skin erythematous or discoloured
- Reduced consciousness.

3 Investigation(s)

- CT nose and para-nasal sinus

- Endoscopic sampling of specimen for confirmation of pathology (Mucorales fungal infection)
- Baseline blood +/- culture of blood and CSF
- Other sites: Broncho-alveolar lavage, skin biopsy.

4 Treatment

- Radical surgical debridement is the mainstay of treatment
- Intravenous antifungal agent eg amphoteracin B
- Correction of underlying risk factors
- Urgent ophthalmic review if eyes involved.

5 Follow-up and additional information

- Soon after discharged from hospital to follow progress of recovery
- High mortality rate (>50%).

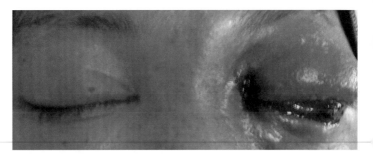

Figure 2.12a Left orbital abscess secondary to mucormycosis.

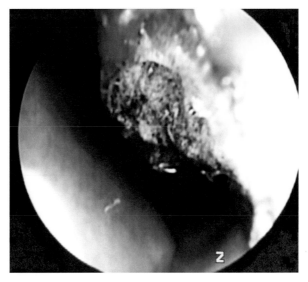

Figure 2.12b Left inferior turbinate involved with mucormycosis.

2.13 BILATERAL CHOANAL ATRESIA

1 History

- A newborn with breathing difficulty, cyanosis but gets pink on crying (suggestive of an upper airway obstruction rather than laryngeal obstruction)
- This is a neonatal emergency so additional information can be gathered later.

2 Examination

- No misting on cold spatula
- No sounds heard with stethoscope under nose
- No success passing a 5F suction catheter through nares after suction and decongestion nasal passage.

3 Investigation(s)

- CT Scan nose and paranasal sinus (especially axial sections) will help to confirm diagnosis (differential diagnosis: bilateral choanal atresia, nasal mass, piriform aperture stenosis, amniotic fluid or severe neonatal rhinitis).

4 Treatment

- Must liase with senior ENT doctor and neonatologist
- Insert Oropharyngeal airway (eg guedal) and secure properly
- Orogastric feeding tube as a neonate is an obligate nasal breather for first 3-6months.
- If bilateral choanal atresia, check for CHARGE (coloboma, heart abnormality, atresia, renal abnormality, genital abnormality, ear abnormality)
- Cardiac ECHO and renal ultra sound scan may be needed and then proceed to surgery
- If piriform aperture stenosis, proceed to surgery
- If nasal mass, refer to appropriate team eg neurosurgeons
- If severe neonatal rhinitis, consider saline douche and diluted decongestants.

5 Follow-up and additional information

- Depending on cause
- Multidisciplinary team
- Neonates are obligate nasal breathers until about 3-6months, this means that they cannot feed and breathe at the same time.

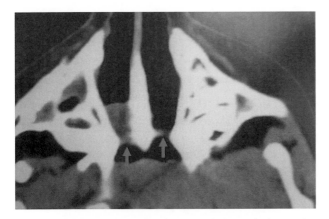

Figure 2.13a Axial CT Scan showing bilateral choanal atresia.

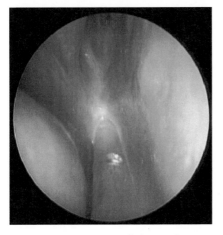

Figure 2.13b Endoscopic view of choanal atresia in the right nostril of a neonate.

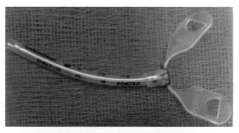

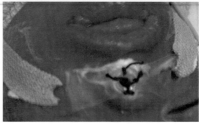

Figure 2.13c Nasal prong for managing nasopharyngeal obstruction of posterior choana is patent (before and after insertion).

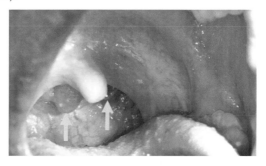

Figure 2.13d Large adenoid causing nasopharyngeal obstruction (tonsils removed already).

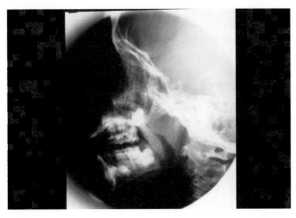

Figure 2.13e Enlarged adenoid blocking the nasopharynx.

2.14 NEONATAL RHINITIS

1 History

- Breathing difficulty improved on crying. Neonates are obligate nasal breathers for first 3-6 months and gross nasal obstruction is life threatening – seek senior input.
- Feeding difficulty
- History of meconium aspiration or maternal genito-urinary tract infection
- No stridor

2 Examination

- Assess for choanal atresia, piriform aperture stenosis or nasal masses.
- Achieved by initial cold spatula mist testing.
- If no mist gently suction the nares with fine tracheal suction catheters.
- If no misting then decongest the nose and gently advance a 5F (1.6mm) suction catheter into the nares to confirm patency of the posterior choanae.
- Examine nose for blue or pale turbinate mucosa associated with thin watery secretion

3 Investigation(s)

- Culture any purulent secretion, especially for Chlamydia.

4 Treatment

- Led by specialist trainee grade in conjunction with neonatologist
- Saline nasal drops and gentle suction.
- Decongestant nasal drops eg diluted xylometazoline hydrochloride for 5/7 maximum.
- Be aware that nasal steroids are not licenced for use in the under 4yrs-olds.

5 Follow-up and additional information

- Ensure follow-up with paediatric ENT team and monitor growth chart and feeding volumes.
- Paediatric allergic rhinitis clinic
- Monitor for eczema, asthma, OME, sinusitis, adenotonsillar hypertrophy

Chapter 3

Throat and Oesophagus

3.1 FOOD BOLUS IN OESOPHAGUS

1 History

- Nature of food bolus
- Time of impaction (sharp bones are emergencies whilst meat bolus may be treated medically for the first 24 hours – see treatment)
- Complete or incomplete dysphagia (increased likelihood of aspiration in complete dysphagia)
- Localisation of level where food bolus appears to be stuck (impaction below the manubrio-sternal angle is more difficult to localised and is best removed by flexible OGD (i.e. gastoenteriology or general surgery)
- Any previous episode.

2 Examination

- Talking in full sentences, regularly spitting saliva into vomit bowl
- Oral and neck examinations are usually unremarkable
- FNE may reveal pooling of saliva.

3 Investigation(s)

- Lateral soft tissue X-ray of the neck to identify a bone or a complication of bone impaction – surgical emphysema or a collection.

4 Treatment

- IV fluids
- IV Buscopan 20 mg every hour for 3 hours, then QDS
- IV prokinetic agent such as Erythromycin (500mg qds) for 24 hours
- If no improvement after 24 hours book patient on the CEPOD list for rigid oesophagoscopy and removal of food bolus
- Post-procedure, start patient on clear fluid first before slowly building up to his or her normal diet prior to discharge
- Monitor for signs of perforation of oesophagus such as neck/back pain on swallowing, increased heart rate, respiratory rate and pyrexia, especially if there were signs of bleeding during endoscopy.

5 Follow-up and additional information

- May need barium swallow to look for stricture as possible cause for bolus impaction
- Refer to gastroenterology if there were signs of oesophageal dysmotility or achalasia.

3.2 FOREIGN BODY IN PHARYNX OR OESOPHAGUS

1 History

- Swallowing of a foreign body
- Dysphagia
- Drooling
- Pain in the throat or behind the sternum
- Regurgitation of food or liquid
- Dysphonia or hoarseness due to laryngeal oedema.

2 Examination

- Foreign body may be seen with FNE
- Localised tenderness in the neck.

3 Investigation(s)

- Lateral soft tissue and anteroposterior X-ray of the neck
- CT scan of the neck

4 Treatment

- Resusitate with IV fluid
- Batteries require urgent retrieval
- Foreign bodies in the pharynx can be removed using appropriate forceps without the need for a GA
- Foreign bodies in the upper oesophagus require removal by an ENT surgeon using rigid oesophagoscopy or removal by a gastroenterologist using flexible oesophagoscopy.

5 Follow-up and additional information

- CT scan may be helpful if the foreign body is easily identified on EUA
- Sharp foreign bodies such as fish bone may get stuck in the tonsil, valleculae, piriform fossa or oesophagus
- Smooth foreign bodies tend to get stuck in the upper oesophagus or at the cardia.

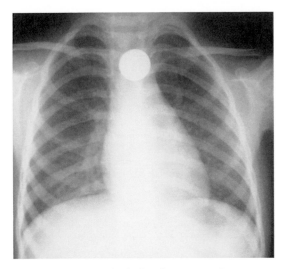

Figure 3.2a Foreign body lodged in cricopharyngeus (level C6).

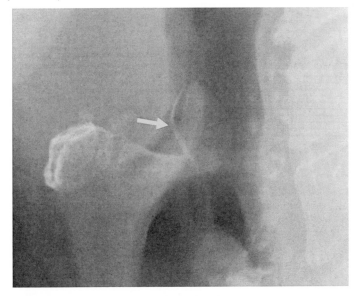

Figure 3.2b Fish bone stuck in the throat.

3.3 TONSILLITIS

1 History

- Odynophagia – duration of symptoms and ability to eat and drink
- Type of analgesia and antibiotics taken
- Frequency of episodes
- Impact on quality of life

2 Examination

- Pyrexia
- Tonsillar exudate and presence of gross hypertrophy with noisy breathing (stertor)
- Grey membrane over tonsil and cervical lymphadenopathy suggests glandular fever
- Trismus and an asymmetrical oropharynx suggest a peri-tonsillar collection (quinsy)
- Symptoms with lack of signs may represent epiglottitis – exclude with FNE

3 Investigation(s)

- FBC including differentials (lymphycytosis and low platelets suggest glandular fever)
- U&Es
- Liver function tests

- Monospot test for Epstein-Barr virus.

4 Treatment

- Admit if unable to take oral antibiotics or fluids
- IV fluids – at resuscitation NOT simply at maintenance rate
- Analgesia – regular paracetamol, NSAID, Difflam spray or gargle
- IV antibiotics (Benzylpenicillin or Clarithromycin)
- Note Amoxicillin or Ampicillin can cause rash with glandular fever
- Dexamathasone may be helpful to reduce swelling in the oropharynx.

5 Follow-up and additional information

- Discharge when able to ear and drink take oral medications
- Scottish intercollegiate guidelines network (SIGN) guidelines suggest tonsillectomy may on balance be appropriate if patients have 7 episodes per year or 5 episodes in 2 years or 3 episodes in 3 years
- Lancefield group A Streptococcal bacteraemia is a Health Protection Association (HPA) notifiable illness
- If Monospot positive, patients have increased risks of hepatosplenomegaly and splenic rupture and should be advised against contact sport and alcohol consumption for at least 4 weeks.

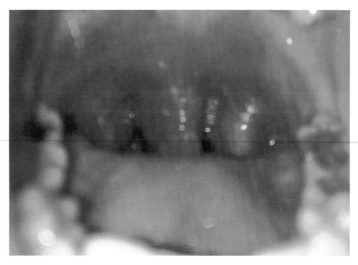

Figure 3.3a Acute bilateral tonsillitis.

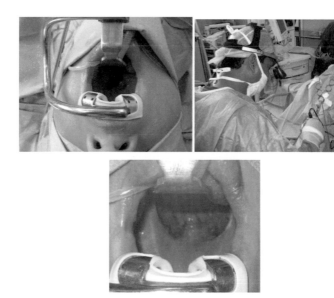

Figure 3.3b-d Tonsillectomy procedure.

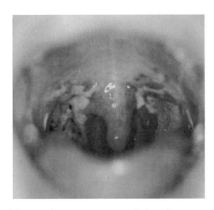

Figure 3.3e Normal appearance of the throat a few days after tonsillectomy.

3.4 QUINSY (PERITONSILLAR ABSCESS) and PERITONSILLAR CELLULITIS

1 History

- History of tonsillitis
- Unilateral sore throat
- Dysphagia
- Otalgia
- Systemically unwell.

2 Examination

- Pyrexia and dehydrated
- Asymmetrical swelling of upper pole of tonsil and soft palate (due to collection of pus outside the capsule) with displacement of the uvula to the opposite side
- Tonsil is pushed downwards and medially
- Trismus – limited jaw opening
- Hot potato voice.

3 Investigation(s)

- FBC, U+Es
- Blood culture if pyrexial
- Monospot test.

4 Treatment

- Aspiration or incision and drainage of abscess under LA
- IV fluids resuscitation and analgesia as per tonsillitis
- Inadequate treatment may result in extensive deep neck space collection – e.g. mediastinal abscess requiring thorocotomy for drainage (Figure 3.4c and d)
- Absence of pus in the peritonsillar region on aspiration could be due to peritonsillar cellulitis or poor technique.

5 Follow-up and additional information

- Patients may benefit from interval tonsillectomy after 2 or more episodes
- Trismus may worsen if aspiration is not performed promptly on admission, making the procedure more difficult.

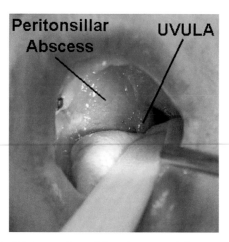

Figure 3.4a Right peritonsillar abscess with associated deviation of the uvula and mild trismus.

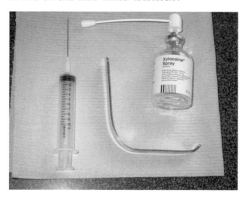

Figure 3.4b Equipment required to aspirate a peritonsillar abscess (LA, Lack tongue depressor, and syringe with a white needle).

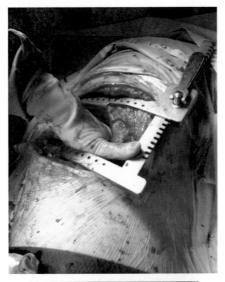

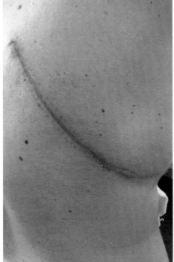

Figure 3.4c & d Thoracotomy to drain a mediastinal abscess secondary to a quinsy (patient lying on his right side) and resulting scar.

3.5 ACUTE EPIGLOTITIS

1 History

- Child 2-4 years old or adult 4th decade
- Sore throat
- Stridor
- Drooling
- Look unwell (toxic)
- Sitting forward (tripod position)
- Differential diagnosis: croup, deep neck space abscess, severe tonsillitis, foreign body impaction.

2 Examination

- Do not examine child but make sure they are in the resuscitation bay of A+E
- Adult may be examined with FNE but certainly not children.

3 Investigation(s)

- None prior to securing the airway
- Then blood culture and microbiology swab of epiglottis.

4 Treatment

- Contact for urgent senior input.
- Upsetting the child may lead to worsening tachypnoea and ventilatory failure. Parents should hold nebulised adrenaline in close vicinity of the child's face (1ml of 1:1000 adrenaline in 3ml saline)
- Calmly transfer the child to theatre for intubation after informing senior paediatric anaesthetist, ENT consultant and theatre staff (diagnosis confirmed by swollen cherry red epiglottis)
- Tracheostomy is rarely required but may be needed if unable to intubate
- Paediatric intensive care unit (PICU) care whilst intubated
- IV antibiotics guided by local protocol
- Repeat laryngoscopy after 48 hours or extubate in the presence of an air leak around the endotracheal tube
- Serological investigations to monitor inflammatory markers.

5 Follow-up and additional information

- No follow-up by ENT required in most cases
- Inspiratory stridor indicates pathology in the supraglottis or glottic regions
- Biphasic stridor indicates pathology in the subglottic or extra-thoracic trachea
- Expiratory stridor (wheeze) indicates pathology in the intra-thoracic trachea and bronchus/lungs.

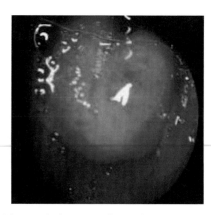

Figure 3.5 Classical cherry red epiglottis seen in acute epiglottis.

3.6 CROUP (LARYNGOTRACHEOBRONCHITIS)

1 History

- Child aged 6 months to 5 years
- Viral inflammation of upper airways, larynx, trachea, bronchi
- Prior subglottic stenosis, previous severe croup and Down's syndrome
- Barking cough
- Hoarse voice
- Coryzal symptoms
- Biphasic stridor, respiratory distress, drooling
- Differential diagnoses – anaphylaxis, inhaled foreign body, epiglottitis, bacterial tracheitis.

2 Examination

- Pyrexia
- Noisy breathing – turbulence at laryngo-trachea manifests as biphasic stridor
- Heart rate, respiratory rate, oxygen saturations on pulse oximetry
- Stridor, nasal flaring, tracheal tug, subcostal recession
- Cyanosis, tracheal tug, subcostal recession and low O2 saturations are late signs
- The absence of stridor may signify exhaustion; associated air movement is now too poor to flow turbulently to create stridor

- Drooling suggests epiglottitis or FB.

3 Investigation(s)

- FBC
- CXR may show Steeple's sign – subglottic oedema (note croup is not in itself an indication for CXR).

4 Treatment

- Supportive
- Nebulised Budesonide and observation

5 Follow-up and additional information

- By paediatrician
- Recurrent, severe or slow to resolve croup may require an elective direct laryngo-tracheoscopy by ENT surgeon to exclude an underlying anatomical abnormality.

3.7 STRIDOR IN ADULT

1 History

- New or progressive – functionally limiting
- Symptoms of sepsis or neoplasia
- Trauma to larynx causing mucosal oedema or haematoma or bilateral cord palsy
- Paradoxical cord movement

2 Examination

- FNE is vital for diagnosis.
- Determine whether stridor is inspiratory, biphasic or expiratory as this indicates the level of obstruction in the airway (Table 3.7).

3 Investigation(s)

- FBC
- Blood culture as appropriate
- Arterial blood gas for CO_2 retention and continuous pulse oximetry.

4 Treatment

- Priority is to determine whether the pathology is progressive and will result in loss of airway and therefore demands early expedited intubation of the airway
- Measures which can be used to 'buy time' before intubation include Heliox (helium 79% oxygen 21%) and nebulised adrenaline (1ml of 1:1000 in 3 ml of normal saline); repeat every 30 minutes if necessary
- IV steroid (6.6mg dexamethasone every 8 hours) and IV antibiotics may reverse the disease process
- Intubation or tracheostomy may be necessary and is best planned by a senior anaesthetist and ENT surgeons.

5 Follow-up and additional information

- Dependant on the cause
- Stridor occurs when 70% of the cross sectional area of the airway has been lost – total respiratory failure may occur very rapidly due to fatigue and CO_2 retention
- Hypoxemia is a late feature.

Table 3.7 Stridor and level of obstruction in the airway

Stridor	Site of obstruction
Inspiratory	Supraglottis Glottis
Biphasic	Subglottis Extra-thoracic trachea
Expiratory (wheeze)	Intra-thoracic trachea Bronchi/alveoli

3.8 VINCENT'S ANGINA

1 History

- Rapid onset of painful bleeding gums
- Poor oral hygiene
- Smoker
- Malnutrition
- Stress
- Immunocompromised

2 Examination

- Poor dentition and oral hygiene
- Bleeding gums

3 Investigation(s)

- FBC
- Smear for fusospirochetal bacteria
- Diagnosis is usually clinical.

4 Treatment

- Admit

- Analgesia and IV fluids for systemic illness
- Antibiotics to cover *Fusobacteria* and *Spirochaete sp* (usually IV metronidazole)
- Improve oral hygiene to prevent recurrence
- Consider debridement of any necrotic areas.

5 Follow-up and additional information

- To prevent recurrence
- Referral to a dentist
- This condition is also known as 'trench mouth' or acute necrotizing ulcerative gingivitis (ANUG)

3.9 ANGIO-OEDEMA

1 History

- Rapid swelling of the skin or mucosa
- Can progress rapidly to an airway crisis
- Ingestion of vaso-dilating foods such as alcohol and cinnamon, may precipitate acquired angio-oedema
- Minor trauma e.g. dental work, may precipitate hereditary angio-oedema; however in most cases the cause is unknown.
- Abdominal pain is associated with hereditary angio-oedema and may mimic appendicitis.

2 Examination

- Stidor
- Signs of anaphylaxis
- FNE to assess upper airway patency.

3 Investigation(s)

- Complement levels - depletion of factors 2 and 4 may indicate C1 inhibitor deficiency
- Serum mast cell tryptase suggests a bradykinin mediated disorder.

4 Treatment

- Call senior anaesthetist and ENT surgeon
- Administer IV antihistamine and steroids with nebulised adrenaline (5ml of 1 in 1000) and high flow oxygen +/- Heliox (79% oxygen, 21% helium) to reduce upper airway resistance.
- N.B. ACE inhibitor induced and hereditary angioedema will not respond to steroids and anti-histamines.
- IV fresh frozen plasma (containing CI-INH) is required for hereditary angio-oedema (CI-INH concentrate is ideal but only available in special centres)
- May require intubation or a tracheostomy to secure the airway.

5 Follow-up and additional information

- Immunology referral for further investigations
- Angio-oedema affects all layers of the skin and mucosa whilst urticaria only affects the upper dermis of the skin
- Essentially the inhibitor of the complement system is deficient or dysfunctional and this result in abnormal activation of the complement system in any part of the body.

3.10 CAUSTIC INGESTION

1 History

- Type, amount and brand name of the ingested material such as bases, acids or bleaches
- Any home treatment used
- Underlying psychological issues
- Chest or abdominal pain
- Hoarseness/stridor
- Dyspnoea
- Odynophagia/drooling.

2 Examination

- Face
- Oral cavity, pharynx and larynx, if possible
- Extremities
- Chest

3 Investigation(s)

- CXR – aspiration pneumonitis, oesophageal perforation and mediastinal widening and infection
- Oesophagoscopy (except in the presence of severe burns with evidence of laryngeal oedema or if patient is on high dose steroids). Timing of EUA is important to minimise risk of iatrogenic perforation.

4 Treatment

- Liaise with senior ENT surgeon and anaesthetist
- Establish likelihood of airway burn or progressive compromise
- Staging oesophagoscopy may be performed - first or second degree burns require antibiotics and steroids along with analgesia and sedation
- Monitor for signs of viscus perforation or sepsis due to trans-mucosal microbiological influx
- Oesophageal stents may be considered by general surgeons
- Button batteriues should be removed immediately and any oesophageal injuries addressed appropriately.

5 Follow-up and additional information

- By MDT to manage aero-digestive strictures
- Investigation into circumstances of ingestion in children or vulnerable adult, by child protection team if deemed appropriate by senior clinician
- Manufacturers and Health and Safety Executive to be informed.

Chapter 4

Neck and Head

4.1 NECK TRAUMA

1 History

- Mechanism of injury - penetrating or blunt trauma
- Symptoms or airway compromise, dysphagia, expectoration of blood or dysphonia.

2 Examination

- As part of a trauma team response - ATLS protocol: ABCDE, primary and secondary survey
- Secure airway and arrest haemorrhage as soon as possible
- Findings demanding emergency EUA include – hypovalaemic shock, rapidly expanding neck haematoma, focal neurology.
- Is there surgical emphysema suggesting injury to larynx/trachea?
- Assessment of the injury location: Is it in Zone 3 (base of skull), Zone 2 or Zone 1 (thoracic outlet)
- Assessment of the depth of injury: has it penetrated platysma? Any obvious structures injured?

3 Investigation(s)

- Bloods including FBC and cross match
- X-rays cervical spine and CXR
- CT angiography of neck to delineate vascular injury if suspected
- Laryngoscopy/bronchoscopy/OGD as guided by patient's symptoms.

4 Treatment

- Involve multiprofessional team (inc. anaesthetist)
- Stabilise C-spine, administer high flow O2, venous access, bloods inc FBC and cross match
- If the patient is unstable (e.g. airway compromise or hypotensive shock unresponsive to resuscitation), urgent surgical exploration is indicated.
- If the patient is stable without signs of obvious vascular injury, and the injury is in zones I or III of the neck, observation may be appropriate.
- If the patient needs surgical exploration for an injury in Zone 1 or Zone 3, CT angiography is necessary because of access to vascular injury is challenging
- Vascular surgery input may be required if large vessels need repair.
- If the patient is stable with a zone II injury, one school of thought advocates surgical exploration if the injury is deeper than platysma. However, this is now becoming less common with CT angiography being the preferred option.

5 Follow-up and additional information

- Long term sequelae of penetrating neck injury may include vascular and neurological complications
- Laryngeal injury can lead to dysphonia
- With regards to cervical trauma, the neck is divided into 3 Zones (Table 4.1). Zone of entry may not represent all zones of injury. Ballistic injury leads to cavitation injury especially if the bullet fragments.

Table 4.1 Traumatic Neck Zones

Neck Zones	Description
1	**From clavicle and sternal notch to cricoid cartilage** • contains arch of aorta, subclavian vessels, thoracic duct, brachial plexus, lung apices • vessels in close proximity to thorax • worse prognosis.
2	**From cricoid cartilage to angle of mandible** • contains common carotid artery and its bifurcations, larynx, hypopharynx, oesophagus, spinal cord, cranial nerves • most commonly involved area, 75%
3	**From angle of mandible to base of skull** • contains interanal carotid artery, external carotid artery, jugular veins, CN VII , pharynx • vessels close to skull base

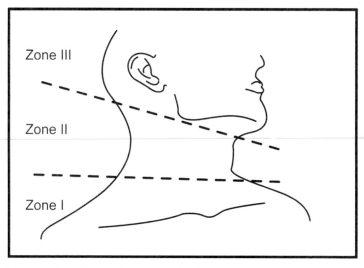

Figure 4.1a Zones in the neck relevant to trauma.

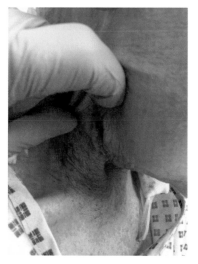

Figure 4.1b Sub-platysmal neck trauma caused by scissors requiring exploration.

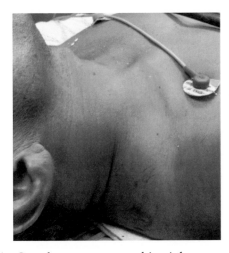

Figure 4.1c Gunshot entry wound in right neck posterior triangle.

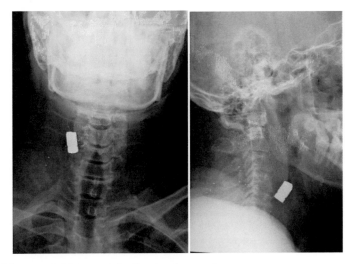

Figure 4.1d & e A bullet in the neck.

4.2 SUPERFICIAL NECK ABSCESS

1 History

- Duration of neck swelling – pre-existing lump, cyst or sinus
- Discharge from abscess
- Systemic illness (fever, malaise) or otherwise well (mycobacterial infection)
- Recent URTI or illness
- Health of other contacts (for child).

2 Examination

- Site, size, fluctuation, overlying skin colour, temperature and pain
- Lymphadenopathy
- General well being (temperature, pulse, BP).

3 Investigation(s)

- Ultrasound scan to help determine the presence of suppuration within a node and need for incision and drainage
- Inflammatory markers +/- blood culture
- Culture/staining of pus if discharging – look for acid fast bacilli.

4 Treatment

- Admit for analgesia and antibiotics
- Antibiotic therapy may be sufficient for small collections with no systemic illness and for mycobacterial illness
- Incision and drainage for simple bacterial infection and biopsy of abscess wall
- Excision for disease suspicious of mycobacterium not responding to antibiotic therapy.

5 Follow-up and additional information

- To assess for residual disease
- Scar assessment

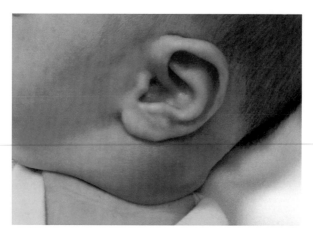

Figure 4.2a Intact superficial neck abscess in a baby.

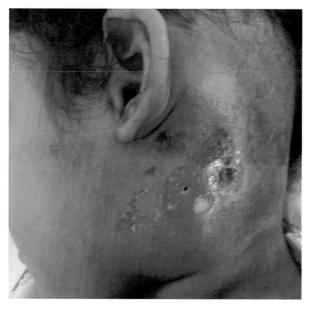

Figure 4.2b Ruptured superficial neck abscess in a child.

4.3 DEEP NECK SPACE INFECTION

1 History

- Painful neck and throat, swelling, swinging pyrexia
- Stridor and drooling
- Reduced range of neck movement
- Preceded by tonsillitis (60%) or dental infection (30%), mastoiditis and pharyngeal foreign body (up to 10% combined). Immune compromised (e.g. diabetes, steroids, disease modifying anti-rheumatic drugs)
- In children, retropharyngeal abscesses may arise after upper respiratory tract infection, tonsillitis, tonsillectomy or foreign body
- In adults, retropharyngeal abscesses may be a rare complication of trauma from septic arthritis or ingested foreign body.

2 Examination

- Airway, breathing and circulation.
- Deep neck space infections may compromise airway by mass effect and circulation from sepsis - seek senior help early and ask for anaesthetic assessment if in doubt.
- Neck examination for masses (parapharyngeal abscesses may be palpable along anterior border of sternocleidomastoid).
- Trismus
- Lateral swelling of the posterior pharyngeal wall

- Marked tenderness on cervical rotation
- Flexible nasendoscopy to visualise airway patency; may also see bulging in lateral or posterior pharyngeal wall.

3 Investigation(s)

- Nasendoscopy to assist assessment for airway compromise
- Blood tests including cultures
- Lateral soft tissue neck x-ray +/- Ortho-pantomogram (OPG) – exclude dental pathology
- CT neck/thorax with contrast to determine nature of infection/abscess, deep neck spaces involved, complications and cause of pathology.

4 Treatment

- Secure airway early (intubation or tracheostomy under local anaesthesia)
- Broad spectrum IV abx pending culture and sensitivity (discuss with microbiologist)
- Incision and drainage (external approach vs per-oral) under general anaesthesia if sign of significant collection or if small collection has not responded to antibiotics or airway is compromised.

5 Follow-up and additional information

- May need elective tonsillectomy or dental extractions dependent on cause
- Common organisms are *Staph aureus* and *Pyogenes* as well as anaerobes
- Complications include mycotic carotid aneurysm, internal jugular vein thrombosis and mediastinitis
- Peak incidence in children is between 1-4 years.

Table 4.3 Prevertebral soft tissue measurements

Vertebrae	Normal width
C1-C4	7mm
C5-T1	17mm

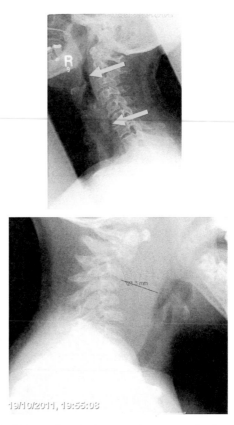

Figure 4.3a Normal and abnormal prevertebral soft tissue swelling.

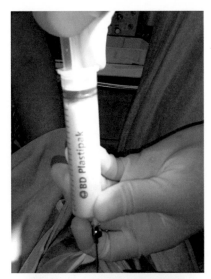

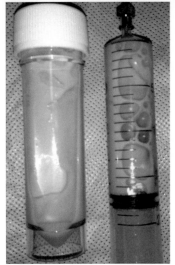

Figure 4.3b &c Aspirating pus from a retropharyngeal abscess in an adult and samples.

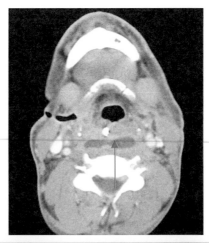

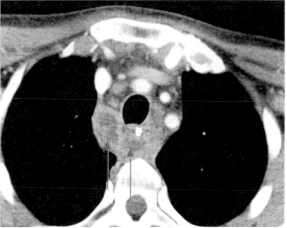

Figure 4.3d&e CT showing a deep neck space abscess with extension into the upper mediastinum.

4.4 LUDWIG'S ANGINA

1 History

- History of tonsillitis (80%) lower molar dental infection (20%)
- Dysphagia (difficulty swallowing)
- Odynophagia (pain during swallowing)
- Difficulty breathing due to swelling in the floor of the mouth
- Immuno-compromised (but can also occur in immunocompetent individuals)
- Recent tongue piercing.

2 Examination

- Pyrexia
- Trismus
- Swollen floor of mouth and submental region due to infection in the sublingual and submandibular spaces
- Stertor due to oropharyngeal obstruction
- FNE to assess upper airway which may be compromised by elevation of tongue and swollen tongue base.

3 Investigation(s)

- FBC
- Blood cultures (usually streptococcus viridan or *E Coli*)
- CT or MRI neck if patient not clinically compromised. OPG (orthopantomogram) to exclude dental pathology

4 Treatment

- Admit (HDU or ITU is ideal) whilst awaiting response to medical therapy or theatre availability
- Analgesia
- Intravenous high dose broad spectrum antibiotics (eg Co-amoxiclav and metronidazole)
- Secure airway with nasopharyngeal intubation or tracheostomy if there is respiratory obstruction
- Incision and drainage of any collection intraorally or externally depending where the infection is localised (sublingual space or submandibular space, respectively).

5 Follow-up and additional information

- Dental referral
- Note that incision and drainage should be postponed until a collection is seen on imaging as pus is rarely found in the early stages.

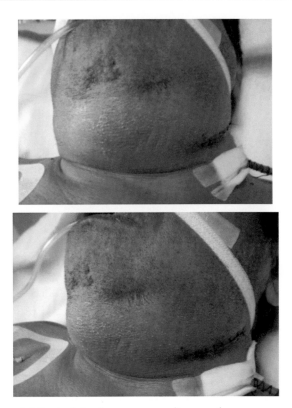

Figure 4.4 Ludwig's abscess extending to the parapharyngeal space.

4.5 LEMIERRE'S DISEASE (Human Necrobacillosis)

1 History

- Patients are usually young healthy adults
- Preceded by a streptococcus sore throat leading to a peritonsillar abscess containing anaerobic bacteria such as *fusobacterium necrophorum*
- Shortness of breath, chest pain and pneumonia due to infected emboli originating from thrombosed internal jugular vein and depositing in the lungs
- Septic shock

2 Examination

- Unwell
- Pyrexia
- Sore throat and parapharyngeal swelling
- Respiratory distress.

3 Investigation(s)

- FBC
- Blood culture +/- joint aspirate culture
- CRP and ESR
- Doppler USS of internal jugular vein but a CT scan or an MRI scan is more sensitive for detecting the thrombus. CT to exclude associated complications.

- CXR

4 Treatment

- Admit
- Analgesia and antipyretics
- Intravenous antibiotics (eg metronidazole and ceftriaxone)
- Incision and drainage of parapharyngeal abscess, if present
- Monitor for septic pulmonary emboli
- Management of internal jugular vein thrombosis is controversial and includes anti-coagulation if signs of propagation and open thrombectomy or ligation.

5 Follow-up and additional information

- To check for any sequelae of the infection or associated disease such as cerebral venous sinus thrombosis or pneumonia.

4.6 CAVERNOUS SINUS THROMBOSIS (CST)

1 History

- Preceding rhinosinusitis
- Preceding preseptal or orbital complications
- Meningism (headache, photophobia, neck stiffness)
- Systemic illness or sepsis
- Other source of infection (teeth, ear).

2 Examination

- Spiking temperature
- Septic
- Nose and sinus examination
- Bilateral eye signs strongly suggest CST incl. proptosis, reduced eye movements, chemosis, reduced visual acuity, altered colour vision)
- Cranial nerves palsy (CN III, IV, V, VI)
- Signs of meningism.

3 Investigation(s)

- CST is a clinical diagnosis.
- CT head with contrast /MR venogram – often a thrombosis is not seen and only indirect signs are present.
- Baseline blood +/- blood culture

- Microbiology swab of any sinus discharge
- +/- Lumbar puncture to rule out meningitis

4 Treatment

- HDU care
- High dose broad spectrum IV antibiotics (discuss with microbiologist)
- +/- Anticoagulant (controversial)
- High dose steroids
- Treat source of infection i.e. sphenoidotomy
- May need surgical decompression of orbital abscess
- Seek ophthalmology and neurosurgical opinion

5 Follow-up and additional information

- May require a prolonged course of antibiotics, even up to 8 weeks so follow up necessary to follow progress of recovery
- Follow up by ophthalmology and or neurosurgery
- Cavernous sinus thrombosis is life threatening with high mortality rate
- Diagnosis is usually clinical
- N.B. chronic inflammatory processes and malignancy may occasionally present as CST.

4.7 SIGMOID SINUS THROMBOSIS

1 History

- Preceding otorrhoea, otalgia, mastoid tenderness and erythema (CSOM)
- Signs of raised intra-cranial pressure (otic hydrocephalus) including – diplopia, altered GCS, blurred vision
- Meningism (headache, photophobia, neck stiffness)
- Sepsis (pyrexia, tachycardia).

2 Examination

- Otoscopy reveals purulent discharge
- Cranial nerve palsy eg VI (lateral rectus palsy)
- Signs of meningism.

3 Investigation(s)

- MR or CT venogram – contrast void with sinus wall enhancement leads to 'delta sign'
- FBC, U&Es, ESR, CRP, clotting profile, blood culture
- Microbiology swab of ear discharge
- +/- Lumbar puncture to rule out meningitis.

4 Treatment

- Management is controversial
- High dose IV antibiotics that crosses blood brain barrier (discuss with microbiologist)
- +/- Anticoagulant
- Treat primary source of infection (eg ear suction clearance)
- Mastoidectomy +/- removal of thrombus +/- ligation of internal jugular vein
- Neurology +/- Neurosurgical opinions.

5 Follow-up and additional information

- Monitor for extension or resolution
- Close follow-up in conjunction with neurology team
- Infection spread from mastoid cavity through emissary veins into sigmoid sinus.

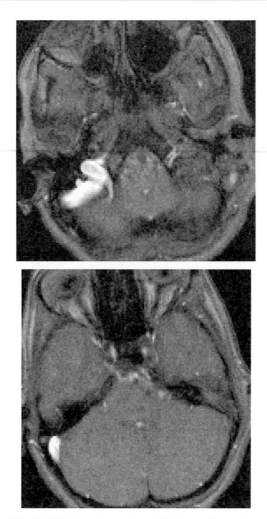

Figure 4.7a MRV showing sigmoid sinus thrombosis (no flow on right side).

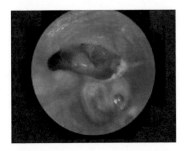

Figure 4.7b CSOM with cholesteatoma is a cause of sigmoid sinus thrombosis.

4.8. ERYSIPELAS

1 History

- Onset, duration, progression, recurrence
- Usually start as a small erythematous patch around nose then rapidly spread outward to the face
- Systemic illness (fever, headache, rigors)
- Immunocompromised, extremes of age, skin trauma.

2 Examination

- Red, painful, shiny, indurated, well-defined/demarcated, flat with raised border lesion in middle third of face
- More advanced infection: Bullae, vesicles, petechiae, necrosis
- Lymphadenopathy

3 Investigation(s)

- Inflammatory markers +/- blood cultures
- Antistreptolysin O titre (Group A Strep).

4 Treatment

- Oral or IV antibiotics (Penicillin/Erythromycin)
- Mark out extent of disease on admission to allow ease of monitoring resolution.

5 Follow-up and additional information

- To assess resolution of symptoms

4.9. CERVICAL NECROTISING FASCIITIS

1 History

- Onset, duration, progression (rapid spreading)
- Source of infection: Skin trauma, preceding deep neck space infections, dental infections, pharyngitis/tonsillitis
- Risk factors: Extreme of age, immunocompromised, uncontrolled diabetes.

2 Examination

- Assess for surgical emphysema and signs of skin necrosis
- Establish extent of pathology and likely surgical teams needed to treat disease process.

3 Investigation(s)

- CT neck (air under skin) and thorax to establish presence of descending mediastinitis
- Blood culture

4 Treatment

- Resuscitation (ABC)
- IV antibiotics (Penicillin and Metronidazole)-
  discuss with microbiologist
- Urgent surgical debridement of necrotic tissue and
  regular reassessments in theatre for further
  debridement, skin grafting, tracheostomy, feeding
  tubes insertion
- +/- Hyperbaric Oxygen therapy (adjunct)
- High mortality rate

5 Follow-up and additional information

- Need to be followed up closely after discharge from
  hospital
- Necrotising fasciitis is bulk tissue necrosis which
  spreads rapidly in the subdermal plane and may be
  under estimated if not actively considered.

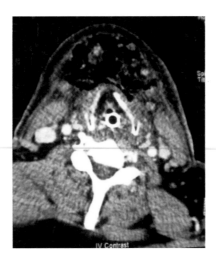

Figure 4.9 Cervical necrotizing fasciitis.

Chapter 5

Complications of Treatment

5.1 ADENOTONSILLECTOMY HAEMORRHAGE (SHOCK)

1 History

- Within the first 24 hours of surgery (primary haemorrhage)
- After 24 hours may be due to infection (secondary bleed)
- Haemoptysis
- Haematemesis
- Coffee-ground vomit, a metallic taste in the mouth, blood stains on pillows

2 Examination

- All post-operative bleeds require readmission
- Attend to patient urgently
- Assess Airway, Breathing and Circulation and make interventions whilst doing so
- Note vital signs, heart rate, respiratory rate, capillary refill time, blood pressure drop is a pre-terminal sign
- Examine oral cavity and note source of bleeding, if

possible
- Note excessive swallowing and anxiousness

3 Investigation(s)

- FBC and U &Es
- Clotting screen
- G&S
- Cross match packed red cells if taking patient to theatre

4 Treatment

- Explain course of action to family and need for resuscitation and observation if stable or EUA
- IV access, if not already present and resuscitate with a bolus of 20ml/kg NaCl stat if child shocked
- Suction any clots in oropharynx and apply adrenaline soaked gauze to tonsil bed if patient allows
- Dilute hydrogen peroxide gargles help remove clots and allow vasospasm (3% hydrogen peroxide gargles in 3 parts water)
- Haemodynamic instability or recurrent paroxysmal heavy bleeds demands EUA
- Patients with minor haemorrhage require admission for close observation for at least 24 hours with IV antibiotics and analgesia; minor haemorrhage may be the sentinel sign for a major bleed

5 Follow-up and additional information

- Screen for Von Willebrand disease and coagulopathy
- Early haemoglobin measurements may under estimate the true volume of blood loss therefore recheck after adequate fluid resuscitation

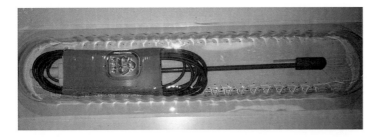

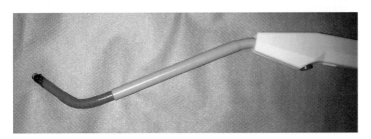

Figure 5.1 a & b Monopolar Suction diathermy (has reduced the incidence of post adenoidectomy bleed from 1.0% to 0.5 %).

5.2 OESOPHAGEAL PERFORATION

1 History

- Recent rigid instrumentation such as oesophagoscopy or endoscopic stapling of pharyngeal pouch
- History of foreign body, penetrating or blunt trauma to the neck, vomiting, malignancy
- Sudden onset interscapular or chest pain
- Note differentials include myocardial infarction, peptic ulcer disease, pneumonia and pancreatitis

2 Examination

- Examination findings may be non-specific or mimic differential diagnoses
- Pyrexia
- Pulse, respiratory rate, blood pressure (shock profile)
- Subcutaneous emphysema
- Interscapular or chest pain

3 Investigation(s)

- FBC, U&E, CRP, LFT, clotting
- Water-soluble contrast studies may demonstrate extravasation of contrast through perforation

- CT scan in patients with suspected mediastinitis, or when contrast swallow studies cannot be performed due to operator or patient factors
- ECG and other investigations relevant to differential diagnoses should be arranged

4 Treatment

- Nil by mouth (NBM)
- IV fluids
- Broad spectrum antibiotics
- Repeat contrast swallow in 7days
- If cervical or thoracic oesophageal leak still present proceed to surgical repair by head and neck surgeon or thoracic surgeon, respectively.

5 Follow-up and additional information

- Water-soluble contrast studies or CT to check for stricture

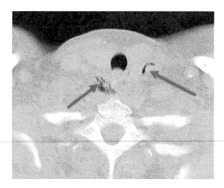

Figure 5.2 CT Scan showing air outside the cervical oesophagus consistent with a perforation.

5.3 POST-THYROIDECTOMY HAEMATOMA

1 History

- Swelling in the neck following thyroidectomy
- Neck pain
- Dyspnoea - due to impaired venous return and secondary laryngeal and tongue base swelling
- Coagulation history

2 Examination

- ABC approach
- Sit patient up
- Assess size and tension of haematoma

3 Investigation(s)

- FBC, clotting screen, Group & Save

4 Treatment

- Mobilise support from anaesthetic colleagues and ENT surgeon
- Administer oxygen via face-mask

- Remove all dressings, sutures or clips to let the haematoma out of the neck aseptically on ward
- Apply pressure to any visible bleeding source
- Return to theatre for arrest of any bleeding vessel, wash out of the haematoma and drain insertion
- Continued airway obstruction (due to tongue base engorgement and laryngeal oedema) may require urgent intubation
- Post-op prophylactic antibiotics

5 Follow-up and additional information

- Check recurrent laryngeal nerve status
- Haematoma may be associated with neuropraxia

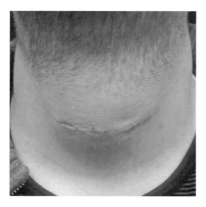

Figure 5.3 Haematoma in the neck after total thyroidectomy.

5.4 HYPOCALCAEMIA FOLLOWING TOTAL THYROIDECTOMY

1 History

- Total thyroidectomy or completion hemi-thyroidectomy performed within last 24 hours
- Documentation of parathyroid glands removed or preserved
- Documentation of central (level 6) cervical lymph node dissection

2 Examination

- Perioral and hand/feet paraesthesia progressing to carpo-pedal spasm
- Laryngospasm – manifest as stridor and respiratory compromise
- Chovstek sign – facial twitching on tapping over the facial nerve in the pre-auricular region inferior to the zygoma

3 Investigation(s)

- Corrected serum calcium, phosphate and magnesium
- Less than 1.8mmol/l ionised calcium is associated with risk of tetany

- ECG to exclude arrhythmia if patient symptomatic or Ca < 1.8mmol/l

4 Treatment

- Admit and then guided by local hospital protocol
- May need to administer 10ml of 10% calcium gluconate by IV infusion as a cardioprotective medication of patient is symptomatic or corrected calcium under 1.8mmol/l in addition to introduction of regular oral elemental calcium. Recheck calcium.
- If persistent hypocalcaemia consider introduction of vitamin D_3
- If still symptomatic re-check Mg – low Mg may have similar presentation to low calcium

5 Follow-up and additional information

- Regular check of ionised calcium
- Twice daily calcium check until stabilised and then weekly until OPD review.
- Total thyroidectomy for Grave's Disease may lead to severe hypocalcaemia secondary to 'hungry bone syndrome' which may take several days to correct.

5.5 FACIAL NERVE PALSY FOLLOWING TYMPANOMASTOID SURGERY

1 History

- Facial palsy following surgery – immediate or delayed
- Check operation notes (usage of nerve stimulator, was facial nerve sacrificed, facial nerve dehiscence, intra-operative bleeding, usage of local anaesthetics)

2 Examination

- Complete or incomplete LMN facial nerve palsy – grade by House-Brackmann scale
- Lacrimation and taste to locate site of nerve injury
- Examine surgical wound for haematoma

3 Investigation(s)

- None in acute setting

4 Treatment

- If you suspect local anaesthesia - wait and recheck

for improvement depending on the LA used

- If you suspect a haematoma - remove bandage and ear packing from mastoid cavity and consider IV steroids
- If a damaged nerve is suspected, surgeon to re-explore with a colleague to assist with repair or nerve grafting
- Delayed facial palsy occurs several days following surgery and may be due to viral reactivation and spontaneously resolves
- Consider oral steroids and eye protection

5 Follow-up and additional information

- Facial palsy often caused by local anaesthesia, bruising to nerve or heating with use of drills and rarely due to transection which is typically complete and immediate
- Delayed and incomplete palsy typically do not require early surgical re-exploration
- May require ophthalmology referral if the eye closure incomplete at 6/52 follow-up
- Dedicated facial physiotherapy may help prevent unhelpful contralateral over compensation

5.6 TRACHEOINNOMINATE FISTULA

1 History

- Tracheostomy (one to two weeks prior)
- Long-term mechanical ventilation
- Neck tumours
- Tracheal surgery

2 Examination

- Brief episodes of bright right red blood peri-tracheostomy site (sentinel bleed)
- Haemoptysis
- Massive peri-tracheal haemorrhage (50% of cases)

3 Investigation(s)

- FBC and U&Es
- G&S or cross match blood

4 Treatment

- Over inflate tracheostomy cuff as most bleeding occur at the level of the endotracheal cuff
- Or replace uncuffed tracheostomy tube with a

cuffed endotracheal tube or cuffed adjustable flange tracheostomy tube, placing the cuff below the site of bleeding to protect the airway and inflate to minimize pulmonary soiling.

- Or use a finger in the airway to compress the innominate artery against the posterior sternum
- Immediate transfer to theatre
- Urgent rigid bronchoscopy, ideally by cardiothoracic team, and direct pressure to tamponade haemorrhage, if necessary
- Median sternotomy and ligation of the innominate artery

5 Follow-up and additional information

- Tracheoinnominate fistula is rare (up to 0.7% associated with tracheostomy) but mortality is approximately 80%
- A sentinel bleed can occur hours to days before the onset of a major haemorrhage
- A high index of suspicion is required for a sentinel bleed in a tracheostomy patient in order to intervene early when the patient is haemodynamically stable

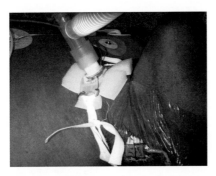

Figure 5.6a An adult patient with an elective tracheostomy for long term ventilatory support (at risk of tracheoinomminate fistula).

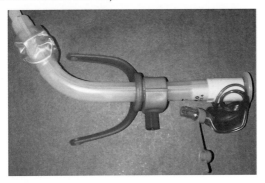

Figure 5.6b Cuffed adjustable flange tube (air is used in cuff).

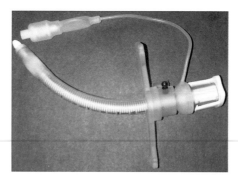

Figure 5.6c Cuffed Bivona tracheostomy tube (water is used in cuff).

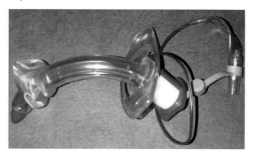

Figure 5.6d Cuffed Portex blue tracheostomy tube.

5.7 CHYLE LEAK

1 History

- Neck dissections or any surgery involving dissection deep to the lower sternomastoid muscle especially in the left supra-clavicular fossa
- Milky fluid is seen in drain bottles following initiation of a fat containing diet
- Occasionally a collection forms in the neck and fistulates through wound dehiscence

2 Examination

- Milky fluid seen in drainage bottle once patient begins to take a diet containing fat
- Intense local inflammatory reaction may result in poor local wound healing
- Profound hypovolaemia, oedema or fluid sequestration, and coagulopathy may occur

3 Investigation(s)

- Diagnosis aided by sample fluid triglyceride level >110mg/dl or greater than serum levels and a protein level >30g/dl – important in equivocal cases as treatment is intensive
- Daily serum electrolytes including Na, K, Ca and

regular albumin, WCC and coagulation screen
- Measuring drain output allows patient categorisation into low flow group <1000ml/day and high flow group >1000ml/day

4 Treatment

- Multidisciplinary team: dietician and pharmacist/clinical biochemist
- Bed rest with meticulous fluid balance, charting and management and daily U&E and replacement
- Conservative treatment for low output leak (<1000ml/day) consisting of an elemental diet with fats restricted to **medium chain triglycerides** only
- Surgical intervention if chronic low output leaks or high volume leaks persists after conservative measure for one week or causing significant compromise
- Somatostatin analogue Octreotide or TPN may also be beneficial
- Early surgical intervention (<1 week post-op) includes local wound exploration, use clips or over-sewing leak with silk suture and local rotation sternomastoid muscle flap (difficult surgery)
- Late surgical intervention (>1 week post-op) is best managed in conjunction with thoracic surgeons and thoracoscopic ligation of the chyle duct - neck exploration at this stage is often highly challenging and unproductive

5 Follow-up and additional information

- Prevention is better than cure
- A rare but potentially life threatening complication following iatrogenic trauma to the thoracic duct
- Loss of fluid, fats, protein, electrolytes and lymphocytes can lead to profound metabolic, immunological and clotting dysfunction with local and systemic wound healing problems
- Chyle fluid production can be between 2 to 4 l/day with the vast majority passing through the thoracic duct
- The thoracic duct typically drains posterior to the left internal jugular vein at its confluence with the subclavian vein but may also empty into the right innominate vein
- Chyle contains lymphocytes, fat soluble vitamins, proteins (30g/dl), electrolytes and breakdown products of long chain fatty acids
- Be aware of the likelihood of delayed local wound healing and infections and the possibility of recurrent leaks following conservative management

5.8 LARYNGECTOMY SPEECH VALVE LEAK

1 History

- Previous laryngectomy with speech valve insertion
- Coughing after eating or drinking
- Weaker voice
- Fluid leaking through valve witnessed by patient in the mirror/ by others at home
- Is the leak through the valve or around the valve?
- When was the valve last changed/replaced?
- Does patient clean the valve regularly?

2 Examination

- Blue-dyed water test-patient swallow and check for leakage either through or around the valve (make sure ready to catch or suck away any leakage of fluid)
- Chest examination - any aspiration pneumonia?

3 Investigation(s)

- FBC, U&Es, CRP
- CXR if suspecting aspiration pneumonia

4 Treatment

- Nil by mouth if come in overnight
- Refer to valve clinic/SALT in the next available slot for replacement of valve
- May need to treat aspiration pneumonia

5 Follow-up and additional information

- Speech valves are usually changed every 3-6 months in OPD
- If speech valve is completely dislodged-secure the tracheo-oesophageal fistula tract with a catheter or NG tube (please familiarize with your local SALT guideline for this situation).

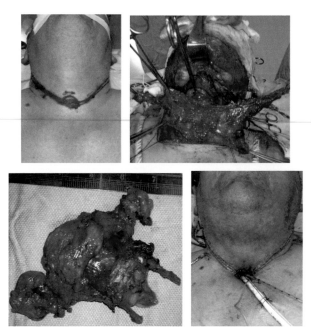

Figure 5.8 Stages in laryngectomy operation (note the blue feeding tube is place in the iatratrogenic tracheo-oesophageal fistula and will later be replaced by a speaking valve.

5.9 RADIATION MUCOSITIS

1 History

- History of head and neck cancer receiving radiotherapy or chemo-radiotherapy
- Sore throat and mouth sores
- Dysphagia and odynophagia
- Nausea and vomiting
- Excessive mucus in mouth/throat or xerostomia
- Weight loss
- Type, duration, dosage and area of treatment received

2 Examination

- Mucosal erythema
- Mucosal exudate
- Confluent ulceration in severe cases
- Assess for dehydration and for cutaneous radiation dermatitis.

3 Investigation(s)

- FBC and U&Es
- Swab mucosa for bacteria and fungi if mucositis excessively severe or extensive for date post radiotherapy

4 Treatment

- Oral care (soft toothbrush, regular rinsing with salt and sodium bicarbonate solution)
- Analgesia – lignocaine gel, gelclair barrier oral gel
- Mouthwash not containing alcohol eg biotene
- Antibiotics/antifungals to be considered if stage of mucositis is out of proportion for that which is expected for the stage post radiotherapy
- May need admission with IV fluids and nasogastric feeding if severe in conjunction with dietician
- Skin care if radiation dermatitis with emollients

5 Follow-up and additional information

- Treatment regime may be interrupted – may need to consult radio-oncologist and MDT
- Early dietitian review especially when patient unable to eat or drink because of mucositis

5.10 BISMUTH IODOFORM PARAFFIN PASTE (BIPP) REACTION

1 History

- Recent history of BIPP pack usage in ear canal or nasal cavity
- Previous exposure to BIPP (more likely to get reaction)
- Duration of contact with BIPP pack (usually reaction starts within 1 week)
- Symptoms of Iodoform reaction (majority): localised dermatitis, itch, pain or more extensive eczema
- Symptoms of Bismuth toxicity: headache, nausea, stomatitis, bismuth line (in gingiva)

2 Examination

- Surrounding skin erythema, oedema and exudate with pruritus and tenderness
- Operative site after removal of pack

3 Investigation(s)

- X-ray if unable to locate pack (BIPP pack normally contain radio-opaque strip)
- +/- patch testing prior to insertion of BIPP pack if

high suspicion of allergy.

4 Treatment

- Removal of BIPP pack following discussion with a senior colleague
- Removal of residual paste
- Analgesia
- Topical steroid cream
- Oral steroid +/- antibiotic, if necessary.

5 Follow-up and additional information

- Check operation site-BIPP reaction may affect outcome of operation requiring revision surgery (for mastoid cavities)
- BIPP is an astringent and antiseptic packing that slowly releases iodine over time
- BIPP reaction is to Iodoform and occurs 48-72 hours after exposure to the antigen
- It is Type IV (delayed) hypersensitivity reaction and therefore involves T cells but no antibodies
- Patients who have been exposed to BIPP are at an increased risk of developing an allergic reaction on second exposure
- Simple alternatives to BIPP include ribbon gauze soaked in steroid/antibiotic creams.

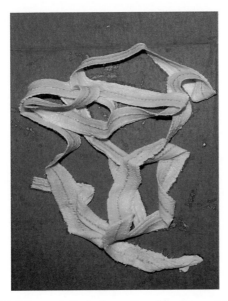

Figure 5.10 Bismuth Iodoform Paraffin Paste (BIPP) packing gauze.

5.11 DRUG INDUCED HEARING LOSS

1 History

- Ototoxic medications e.g. aminoglycoside antibiotics (most cochleotoxic is Neomycin followed by Amikacin and Kanamycin); note that gentamicin is more vestibulotoxic than cochleotoxic
- Loop diuretics, quinine, heavy metals and chemotherapeutic agents (salicylates causes reversible tinnitus only)
- FH of ototoxicity
- Vertigo (ototoxic medications are often vestibulotoxic)
- Co-existing renal dysfunction which prevents elimination of ototoxic drugs.

2 Examination

- Otoscopy normal
- Nystagmus due to associated vestibulo-toxicity.

3 Investigation(s)

- Pure tone audiometry reveals sensori-neural hearing loss
- If FH of aminoglycoside sensitivity should consider genetic referral for exclusion of A1555G

mitochondrial mutation inherited through the maternal line.

4 Treatment

- Stop the offending drug if the clinical condition permits
- Consider an alternative medication
- Amplification may be required to improve the hearing
- In the vast majority of cases, once the ototoxic drug is withdrawn, the hearing will return to normal within a few days
- Hearing aids may be required if hearing loss remains significant
- If air conduction hearing aids are inadequate and profound senori-neural hearing loss is bilateral, then consider referring for cochlear implant MDT assessment.

5 Follow-up and additional information

- Serial PTAs
- Ototoxicity is defined as a greater than 10dB reduction in hearing at one or more bone conduction frequency bilaterally; it most commonly affects high frequencies initially, progressing to involve the lower frequencies.
- It is important to exclude other causes of sensorineural hearing loss in these patients, and

investigate accordingly
- Ototoxic drugs leach into the endolymph of the inner ear and cause direct damage to the outer hair cells initially and later the inner hair cells
- Damage can also occur to the vestibular apparatus
- The cochlear hair cell damage may be due to free-radical damage from reactive oxygen species as a result of the drug action

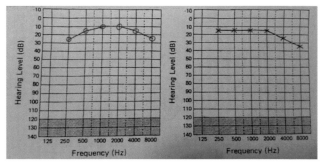

Figure 5.11a Audiogram of a patient at the start of Amikacin for resistant tuberculosis.

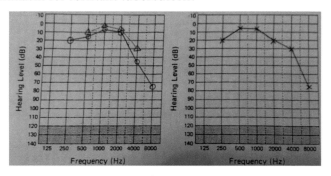

Figure 5.11b Audiogram of the same patient one month later showing sensorineural hearing loss.

5.12 BAHA INFECTION

1 History

- Discharge around abutment site is a common complication
- Localised discomfort or pain
- Implant loosening
- Date of implantation
- Routine follow-up clinic date.

2 Examination

- Remove, or ask the patient to remove the BAHA sound processor - you might now see the abutment
- Be familiar with what a healthy BAHA abutment site looks like (see photo)
- Note any discharge or soft tissue over-growth
- Varying degrees of skin reaction in increasing severity - from erythema, swelling, moistness, granulation tissue to extrusion
- The abutment or implant may not be visible in severe infection where either it has extruded, or overgrowth of granulation tissue has occluded it from view.

3 Investigation(s)

- Swab discharge
- Review *methicillin resistant staphylococcus aureus* (MRSA) carriage status.

4 Treatment

- Outpatient-based care (the patient will often be expert in managing such episodes)
- Spray abutment site with local anaesthetic spray
- Gently remove any debris accumulating between abutment and soft tissue interface with Jobson-Horne probe (flat end)
- Topical therapy (e.g. fucidin HC or otocomb ointment) applied to abutment site TDS for 5/7
- Oral therapy with skin commensal cover if no response to local therapy
- If soft tissue overgrowth prevents the processor clipping consider leaving the aid off to minimise repeated trauma
- Occasionally it is necessary for the patient to require soft tissue excision in theatre or the removal of the abutment to allow tissue overgrowth followed by re-punch and reattachment of the abutment
- Tightening of loose abutments using appropriate equipment.

5 Follow-up and additional information

- BAHAs are 'bone anchored hearing aids'. Implanted either for a conductive hearing loss with inability to wear conventional hearing aid OR unilateral dead ear.
- Comprise a simple 4mm titanium implant drilled into the skull cortex behind the pinna attached to a fixed trans-cutaneous abutment (i.e the pin) which the small box hearing aid clips to
- DO NOT CONFUSE BAHA WITH A COCHLEAR IMLPANT
- Historically implanted into skull having removed the overlying scalp soft tissue and hair with resultant bald depression to scalp. New types are simply implanted through a skin punch.
- To prevent complications, advise patients of meticulous BAHA care, particularly in the early post-operative period

- Ensure follow-up in BAHA clinic <2/52. Be aware that without the implant the patient may be left profoundly handicapped. Liaise with BAHA audiologist for loan of BAHA soft band.

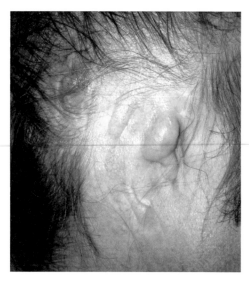

Figure 5.12a. Infected BAHA site in a patient with Type IV Microtia (or Anotia).

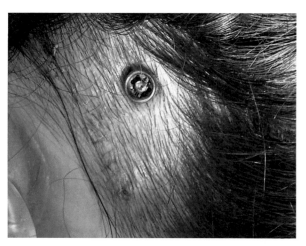

Figure 5.12b An implanted titanium BAHA long stem abutment screw which reduces skin complications.

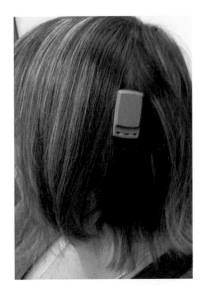

Figure 5.12c A BAHA processor attached to abutment screw.

5.13 COCHLEAR IMPLANT INFECTION

1 History

- When was the implantation surgery performed?
- Symptoms of middle ear infection versus receiver package infection?
- Signs of meningism?
- Vaccination history and history of chronic middle ear disease
- Type of device implanted – spacer used (1999-2002)
- History of inner ear malformation e.g. Mondini malformation

2 Examination

- Cochlear implant comprises a transmitter coupled magnetically to a sub-galeal receiver unit sited above and behind the pinna connected to an electrode which runs into the middle ear and cochlea
- External examination for fluctuant or tender swelling to the receiver site having asked the patient to remove the external processor
- Dehiscence of post-aural wound or extrusion of the receiver package through the overlying skin flap
- Otoscopy for signs of acute otitis media (AOM)
- Neurological examination, GCS and signs of meningeal irritation

3 Investigation(s)

- Swab any pus in ear canal and review MRSA carriage status
- Baseline inflammatory markers – FBC and CRP
- Contact the cochlear implant centre to establish the type of implant used.

4 Treatment

- Must liaise with senior ENT trainee and cochlear implant centre and MDT
- **Acute otitis media** – can lead to meningitis especially if within 2 months of implantation or if spacer device used to fix electrode to cochlea. There is no role for simple supportive treatment – all patients should receive antibiotics and monitor for signs of meningitis. If <2/12 post implantation – admit for IV cephalosporin antibiotics with CNS penetrance. If >2/12 post-implantation and not systemically unwell, without spacer device or inner ear malformation can treat with oral therapy and close observation.
- Receiver site infections should be treated with IV antibiotic therapy to cover *Staph aureus*. If signs not resolving may require receiver site washout or device explantation.

5 Follow-up and additional information

- Patients are profoundly hearing impaired without the device. Most children will however have bilateral implants.
- All patients undergoing implantation should have received vaccination against common bacterial infections causing AOM including *Haemophilus influenza* type B, polyvalent pneumococcal and meningococcal vaccines
- Most receiver site infection occurring under 1year post-op may be due to bacterial inoculation at the time of surgery
- Early follow-up must be arranged with the cochlear implant MDT.

5.14 CAROTID BLOWOUT

1 History

- Primary diagnosis and prognosis including the presence of a 'Do Not Attempt Resuscitate (DNAR)' order
- Date and nature of surgery
- Post-operative adjuvant chemo- or radiotherapy
- Volume of bleeding from neck, pharynx or laryngectomy stoma and frequency
- Does the patient have 1) local recurrence with fungating tumour, 2) post-op with salivary fistula from pharynx or 3) post radiotherapy.

2 Examination

- Must rapidly stabilise the patient whilst examining including airway protection
- Determine site of bleeding and estimate blood volume loss
- Is the patient haemodynamically decompensating and if for active treatment do they need to be transferred to a site for aggressive resuscitation e.g. theatre recovery.

3 Investigation(s)

- FBC, coagulation screen.
- If patient is stable contact interventional radiology to help establish and treat the source of the bleed.

4 Treatment

- C then ABC. Firm pressure over the source of bleeding and two wide-bore IV cannula. Cuffed tracheostomy tube should be inserted into the laryngectomy stoma to minimise pulmonary soiling.
- Activate the 'major haemorrhage protocol' through the transfusion service to obtain 4 units of Group O –ve packed red cells and FFP. Coagulation screen and monitor for side effects of massive transfusion.
- Urgent assessment by senior anaesthetist and ENT surgeon to determine if and where treatment should occur and a senior radiologist
- If patient is stable and able to lay flat alone CT imaging can help guide the surgeon toward the exact source of bleeding.
- Only palliate if there is documented evidence of this decision – until senior review
- Follow local protocol which may include the use of a midazolam syringe driver to control patient anxiety, if appropriate.

5 Follow-up and additional information

- Small volume bleeds can be 'herald bleeds' prior to a major blow out
- Sentinel bleeding must be taken seriously and seen as an opportunity to determine the appropriateness of active treatment in the event of a large blow out or intervene to correct provoking factors e.g salivary fistula, local wound infection, exposed great vessels
- Methods of controlling a blow-out include endoluminal stenting by an interventional radiologist with the risk of future stent infection if the patient is stable
- Common or internal carotid artery ligation which carries a CVA and mortality risk
- Internal jugular blow out may also lead to rapid exsanguination.

Glossary

AC – air conduction

ARS – acute rhinosinusitis

AOM – acute otitis media

BAHA – bone anchored hearing aid

BC – bone conduction

BIPP – bismuth iodoform paraffin paste

BPPV – benign paroxysmal positional vertigo

CN7 – 7th cranial nerve i.e. facial

CSF – cerebrospinal fluid

CT – computed tomography

CNS – central nervous system

CRP – c reactive protein

CSOM – chronic suppurative otitis media

CST – cavernous sinus thrombosis

CXR – chest x-ray

CVA – cerebrovascular accident

DH – drug history

EAC – external auditory canal

EUA – examination under anaesthesia

FB – foreign body

FBC – full blood count

FH – family history

G+S – group and save

GA – general anaesthetic

GCS – Glasgow coma scale

FNE – flexible nasendoscopy

HDU – high dependency unit

HHT – hereditary haemorrhagic telangiectasia

HPA – Health Protection Agency

ICP – intracranial pressure

IV – intravenous

ITU – intensive care unit

LMN – lower motor neurone

MC&S – microscopy culture and sensitivity

MDT – multidisciplinary team

MR – magnetic resonance

MS – multiple sclerosis

NAI – non-accidental injury

NBM – nil by mouth

OPD – outpatient department

PICU – paediatric intensive care unit

PTA – pure tone audiogram

SIGN – Scottish intercollegiate guidelines network

SSNHL – sudden sensorineural hearing loss

TIA – transient ischaemic attack

TM – tympanic membrane

U + Es – urea and electrolytes

UMN – upper motor neurone

URTI – upper respiratory tract infection

Request from the authors

There is always room for improvement and therefore we would be very grateful for your constructive feedback and comments on the content of this book.

Please send your feedback via email to info@enttzar.co.uk or ricardopersaud@yahoo.co.uk.

You may also wish to review this book on Amazon.

Your comments are important to us as we think about improvements for the 2nd edition.

Many thanks
RP, SF, MK, EW & YB
www.enttzar.co.uk